THE T

Lifestyle ha
jumpstart your energy, boost y__   *d*
enhance your manhood.

By Damon J. Smith

NOTE: The contents of this book are intended for informational and educational purposes only, and are not intended to replace a doctor's medical advice. This book should not serve as a substitute for professional medical advice, diagnosis or treatment. Always seek the advice of your physician or other qualified health care provider with any questions you may have regarding your medical condition. Never disregard professional medical advice or delay seeking it because of something you've read in this or any other book.

With that said, you do have the right to seek out a second opinion, find a qualified medical practitioner who utilizes natural and complementary medical treatments, and make your own choices for your body!

As we age, men's testosterone levels decline gradually, a phenomenon known as "andropause." It contributes to a decline in sex drive, decreased muscle mass, hair loss, weight gain, loss of energy, and sometimes moodiness. Although it's a natural part of aging, unhealthy aspects of today's modern culture may actually lower testosterone levels prematurely, leading to a condition called "hypogonadism."

According to the Urology Care Foundation,

> "Roughly 40% of men with high blood pressure will have low testosterone levels. Additionally, approximately 50% of men with diabetes and 50% of obese men will have low testosterone."

Although conventional medicine may call for testosterone replacement therapy in the form of pharmaceutical drugs as the solution to this problem, fortunately it's not difficult to increase testosterone naturally.

These 16 keys for increasing testosterone will require some lifestyle changes, but the good news is that these are the very changes that will not only boost your testosterone, but they will also help you enjoy improved overall health and quite possibly prevent or combat chronic illness.

1. Sleep

In one study, researchers at the University of Chicago found that young men who slept less than five hours a night for one week had lower testosterone levels than when they were fully rested. Sleep deprivation affected their testosterone levels by as much as 10-15% . Try to get at least 7-9 hours of sleep every night.

If you have trouble getting to sleep or staying asleep through the night, try eliminating any sources of artificial light that may be entering your room. Invest in some blackout shades, move your alarm clock to a nearby room, and make sure the TV and/or other electronics are turned off when you go to sleep. If possible, stay away from your smartphone, tablet, computer, TV and other electronics for at least an hour before bedtime, as these stimulants can disrupt your energy levels and contribute to restlessness.

If you're mind is "busy," try reading a book, listening to music, or solving a puzzle before going to bed.

2. Lose Weight

Losing the excess pounds may increase your testosterone levels. Removing fast food, highly processed foods and soda from your diet is critical. It's especially important to remove any foods or drinks that contain high fructose syrup, aspartame, sucralose, saccharin, neotame, and other artificial sweeteners.

High insulin levels contribute to low testosterone, and testosterone levels decrease after you eat sugar. Refined carbohydrates like breakfast cereals, bagels, waffles, pretzels, and most other processed foods also quickly break down to sugar, increase your insulin levels, and cause insulin resistance, which is the number one underlying factor of nearly every chronic disease and condition known to man, including weight gain. Overall, losing weight is a great start to boosting your testosterone levels.

3.   Do Short Periods of High-Intensity Exercise or Interval Training

Bouts of short intense exercise have been shown to boost testosterone and prevent its decline. That's unlike aerobics or prolonged moderate exercise, which have shown to have negative or no effect on testosterone levels.

1. Do a 3 to 5 minute warm up
2. Stretch your body for 1-2 minutes
3. Exercise as hard and fast as you can for 60 seconds. You should feel like you couldn't possibly go on another few seconds
4. Recover at a slow to moderate pace for 60 seconds
5. Repeat the high intensity exercise and recovery 5 more times

Note that the entire workout is only 15-20 minutes. Twenty minutes a day of focused, high intensity exercises is really all you need! Try this on a rower, bike, or circuits with weights and plyometrics are also great high intensity workouts for those who are more advanced.

4. Consume Plenty of Zinc

The mineral zinc is very important for testosterone production. Research has shown that restricting dietary sources of zinc leads to a significant decrease in testosterone, while zinc supplementation increases and even protects men from reductions in testosterone levels. If you have low testosterone levels, you may see improvement in as little as six weeks simply by adding zinc to your diet.

We always recommend incorporating vitamins and minerals in the diet naturally, through whole foods, as most commercial supplements never get absorbed into the bloodstream. You can spend a pretty penny on some of those supplements, only to find them washed down the urinal! Eating them in a well balanced diet is not only more effective, but it's also much more enjoyable. Foods high in zinc include oysters, grass fed beef and lamb, wheat germ, spinach, raw pumpkin seeds, raw cashews, pastured pork and chicken, beans and mushrooms.

5. Reduce Stress

When you're under a lot of stress, your body releases high levels of the stress hormone cortisol. This hormone blocks and limits testosterone production.

High levels of cortisone in men also contributes to fatigue, depression, weight gain, bone and muscle loss, foggy thinking, anxiety and irritability. It breaks down muscle, slows the immune system, and in the process, lowers your testosterone levels.

One of the best ways to regain balance with cortisol levels is to get more sleep. Another is to incorporate regular bursts of high intensity exercise into your daily routine (studies actually show that working out at the gym, excessive cardio and strength training may actually increase cortisol levels). If you can improve your sleep, diet and exercise for at least a month, you will find your cortisol levels fall right in line and your whole body will show major improvements.

6. Eat Healthy Fats

By healthy, this means not only mono- and polyunsaturated fats, like that found in avocados and nuts, but also saturated, as these are essential for building testosterone. Research shows that a diet with less than 40 percent of energy as fat (and that mainly from animal sources, i.e. saturated) may lead to a decrease in testosterone levels.

Examples of healthy fats you can eat more of to give your testosterone levels a boost include:

- Olives and cold pressed olive oil
- Coconuts and cold pressed virgin coconut oil
- Butter made from raw grass-fed organic milk
- Raw nuts, such as, almonds or pecans
- Organic pastured egg yolks
- Avocados
- Grass-fed meats
- Palm oil
- Unheated organic nut oils

7. Power of the Mind

Believe you are strong, vibrant and vigorous! Affirm yourself daily and you will take the proper actions to create the mind, body and soul you want. If you struggle in this area, check out www.Soulpower.Academy, our 40-day mental transformation program.

8. Benefits of Squats: Total Body Exercise

Squats help to build your leg muscles that includes your quadriceps, glutes, hamstrings, and calves, but they also create an anabolic environment, which promotes body-wide muscle building. When squats are performed intense enough they trigger the release of testosterone. Squats help you improve both your upper and lower body strength due to the fact it takes entire body control to do a proper squat.

9. Vitamin D Supplementation - Vitamin D deficiency is a growing epidemic in the US, and is profoundly affecting men's health. The cholesterol-derived steroid hormone vitamin D is crucial for men's health. It plays a role in the development of the sperm cell nucleus, and helps maintain semen quality and sperm count.

The number one best way to improve vitamin D levels is to get more sun exposure. Depending on the time of the year and your pigmentation, as little as 10-20 minutes of sunlight each day –

preferably exposing as much skin as possible to the sun – can increase your vitamin D levels. Ideally, you want to stay in the sun just long enough to begin to bring color to your skin and generate a little sweat. Do not stay long enough to burn your skin, and be careful not to wash the oils from your skin for an hour or so. The point is to allow the oil in your skin to convert the sunlight into vitamin D.

Vitamin D supplements may be an option, but most are synthetic forms of vitamin D, and your body knows the difference and will only use a small portion of synthetic vitamins. If you live in an area with little sunlight, the best option for supplementation is a high quality cod liver oil. A high quality cod liver oil provides both vitamin A and D at levels that complement one another; however, low quality cod liver oil may be deficient in vitamin D and should be avoided. Visit our page dedicated to cod liver oil for recommendations of the best brands to choose: www.souleticsresourcecenter.com/super-food-supplement-cod-liver-oil.

10. Phosphatidylserine (PtdSer or "PS")

Phosphatidylserine is a phospholipid, a naturally occurring amino acid present in the inner leaflet of the cell membrane of almost all of the cells of our bodies. Its main function is to deliver bodily signals between cells and hormones, but it can also reduce oxidative stress, reduce inflammation in the body, improve the testosterone to cortisol ratio, promote DHT turnover, and even improve cognitive functions.

The majority of research pertaining to PtdSer revolves around memory and cognitive function. However, a small number of peer reviewed research indicates that 750-800 mg/day of PtdSer combined with exercise can reduce cortisol levels, especially in response to exercise induced oxidative stress. So, in laymen's terms, if you're a workout fanatic, a high quality supplement of "PS" may be in order. Otherwise, good whole food sources of PtdSer include tuna, pastured chicken, organ meats, such as beef or chicken liver, and white beans.

11. Creatine

Creatine is a natural substance that is present in almost all vertebrates, which helps supply energy to muscles and all cells throughout the body. It's a key component in skeletal muscle metabolism, and it's also the most researched and respected bodybuilding supplement out there.

One highly referenced study on creatine showed that men who rigorously trained while supplementing with creatine reflected a significant increase of testosterone levels. Their T levels were also higher than other men who rigorously trained but took a placebo instead of creatine.

While supplementing with creatine is generally considered safe when following dosage recommendations (excessive creatine may stress the kidneys), it is also easy to get in whole food sources. Organ meat is by far the best food source of creatine, as are pastured beef and poultry, and wild or sustainably farmed fish. However, creatine breaks down under high heat levels, so you must either consume raw meat (which we do not recommend), or slow cook it at low temperatures. You will find some great slow cooker recipes in later chapters.

12. High Quality Organic Foods

Foods that have not been treated with pesticides not only are free from the toxic load of those poisons, but numerous recent studies have revealed that organic foods have more antioxidants and micronutrients than conventional foods. One theory states that organic plants develop chemicals to protect themselves from pathogens, and when we consume those plants we reap the benefit of those chemicals fighting off pathogens in our bodies, as well. These pathogen fighting substances are not found in conventional plants that rely on pesticides to do the work for them. Regardless of "why" organic plants have more cancer fighting compounds like antioxidants and polyphenols, the research shows they are far superior to conventional foods.

Additionally, many of the pesticides, insecticides, herbicides and fungicides sprayed on conventional foods contain anti-androgens, which are chemicals known to block androgen production and receptor activity.

IMPORTANT THINGS TO AVOID

Dr. Mercola, who maintains the #1 ranked health resource

website, outlines four important things to avoid that have a negative impact on your testosterone:

13. Avoid Commercial Dairy Products that contain Bovine growth hormones.

These are Estrogen-mimicking and growth-promoting chemicals that are typically added to commercial dairy products.

14. Avoid Unfermented Soy Products

Soy contains anti nutrients and hormone-like substances, and is NOT a health food (contrary to popular belief). The only way to enjoy soy is by traditional fermentation methods, such as a traditionally fermented soy sauce (which must be specifically sought out, as most commercial brands of soy sauce found in the U.S. are not fermented). Visit this page on Mercola's site to learn more about the dangers of soy: soy.mercola.com

15. Avoid MSG

Monosodium Glutamate is a dangerous food additive that improves the taste of cheap foods, but can negatively impact reproductive health and fertility. MSG is also a known carcinogen, meaning it is known to cause cancer.

16. Avoid Fluoride

A potent neurotoxin found in most U.S. water supplies, fluoride is linked to endocrine disruption, decreased fertility rates, and lower sperm counts. Invest a little extra time and money to locate a water filter that specifically filters out fluoride. Also, non fluoridated toothpaste is a good option. I've been using non-fluoridated toothpaste for about 5 years now and I've found those brands to be far superior to commercial brands of fluoridated toothpaste.

CHAPTER 2: The Importance of Sleep

Healthy sleep patterns are incredibly important for overall well being, and even more important for maintaining optimal testosterone levels. Almost all living beings have an internal "circadian clock" that regulates the timing periods of sleepiness and wakefulness throughout the day, with "circadian rhythms" that dip and rise at different times of the day. Maintaining a consistent sleep/wake restorative process (i.e. getting a good night's sleep regularly), will help keep your circadian clock in balance and eliminate the any intense sleepiness you may encounter in the afternoon.

In one study, researchers gathered a group of healthy men to test their T levels upon waking. The men who had slept for 4 hours showed T levels of 200-300ng/dl, whereas the men who slept for 8 hours showed T levels of 500-700ng/dl, demonstrating a direct link between length of sleep and testosterone levels. A similar study showed that men who slept 4 hours a night had T levels of 60% less than men who slept 8 hours a night. The results of both studies indicate that simple sleep is enough to boost testosterone!

Your testosterone levels follow a circadian rhythm, peaking in the morning and slowly declining towards the evening. Even in your sleep, your body follows a rhythm, cycling between REM (Rapid Eye Movement) and non-REM sleep. The REM stages of sleep is when dreams occur. When you're in the REM stages of sleep, your eyes move rapidly and your brain functions similarly to the way it functions when you are awake, only your body is temporarily paralyzed, which is why you don't act out your dreams. If you find yourself thrashing wildly, talking or otherwise acting out your dreams, this is a sign of REM sleep deprivation.

During the REM stages of sleep, it is normal for your penis to become erect. In fact, during a normal night of sleep the penis may be erect for a total time of from one hour to as long as three and a half hours during the total combined periods of REM sleep. If you suffer from erectile dysfunction while awake, but achieve erections in your sleep, it may indicate that the dysfunction stems from a psychological cause. Nevertheless, during REM stages of sleep your body produces ample amounts of testosterone, so it goes without saying that REM sleep is critically important to boosting testosterone levels.

Typically, REM sleep occurs 90 minutes after you fall asleep, with the first cycle lasting about 10 minutes. Each REM cycle that follows lasts longer, with the final REM stage lasting up to an hour. Since your body cycles through 3 additional stages of Non-REM sleep throughout the remaining hours of the night, during which time the body repairs and regrows tissues, builds bone and muscle, and strengthens the immune system (when the bulk of your naturally occurring Human Growth Hormone, or HGH, is produced), it's important to give your body enough total hours to complete each cycle completely and restfully. Just a few additional hours of sleep each night can literally double your testosterone levels!

The Many Ways Disrupted Sleep Patterns Can Impact Your Health

If you're unable to get enough hours of sleep on a regular basis, or if you're constantly waking up throughout the night, it won't take long for you to notice the ill consequences. These are some of the negative repercussions that follow lack of sleep.

Short term memory

Your circadian clock controls your daily cycle of sleep and wakefulness by alternately regulating the release of certain neurotransmitters, which inhibit and excite different parts of your brain. The part of your brain known as the hippocampus must be excited in order for the things you learn to be organized in such a way that you'll remember them later.

If your internal clock isn't functioning properly, it causes the release of too much Gamma-Amino Butyric Acid (GABA). While GABA inhibits nerves in an effort to calm nervous anxiety, an excess of GABA inhibits your brain in a way that can lead to short term memory problems and the inability to retain new information.

Creativity and learning performance

Proper sleep enhances performance, learning and memory by improving your creative ability to uncover new connections among seemingly unrelated ideas.

Weight gain/loss

Lack of sleep affects levels of metabolic hormones that regulate feelings of hunger and fullness. For example, leptin, the hormone that tells your brain your stomach is full, decreases when you are sleep deprived. Simultaneously, levels of ghrelin, a hormone that triggers hunger, increases with sleep deprivation.

Immune system

Research has found that when you are well-rested you are likely to have a stronger immune response to viruses than when you have not gotten enough sleep. It's believed that the release of certain hormones during sleep is responsible for boosting your immune system.

Stress

Disruptions in your circadian cycle may also raise your levels of the stress hormone cortisol. This hormone increases your heart rate and blood pressure, which can turn every day annoyances into triggers for intense anger. When your body experiences stress, your muscles tense up, your digestion slows, and your brain chemistry changes. Over time, consistently high levels of cortisol can lead to serious health problems, weight gain, and low testosterone.

Chronic Illness

According to numerous studies, including a report in the *Journal of the American Medical Association* (JAMA), lack of sleep can cause or further exacerbate other serious and chronic diseases, including:

- Cancer
- Type 2 Diabetes
- Coronary Heart Disease
- Parkinson Disease
- Alzheimer Disease
- Multiple Sclerosis
- Gastrointestinal Tract Disorders

- Kidney Disease
- Behavioral problems in children

Natural Ways to Regulate your Circadian Clock

It may seem overly simple, but the most effective way to maintain a natural circadian rhythm is to manage your exposure to light and darkness. Humans need regular exposure to bright light during the day and absolute darkness while we sleep at night, but many of us work in poorly fluorescent lit office environments and go home in the evening to excess light stimulation.

If you can control your office environment, invest in some full-spectrum light bulbs that mimic the spectrum of light found in outdoor environments. If you cannot control your lighting, then go outside as much as possible throughout the day and, if possible, seat yourself indoors near a window with exposure to plenty of natural light.

In your home, you might consider installing "low blue" bulbs that emit an amber light in order to minimize evening exposure to melatonin suppressing blue light. TV and computer screens also emit blue light, so you should try to turn those off in ample time before bed – if possible, as soon as the sun goes down.

Then, once you retire to the bedroom, try to make it as dark as possible – like so dark you can't see your hand in front of your face. Even small amounts of light can be enough to suppress melatonin production for that sleep cycle, so do your best to keep from getting up and turning on bathroom or hallway lights in the middle of the night. If you can't get your room dark enough with blackout shades or heavy drapes, it may be a good idea to buy a good quality eye mask to wear through the night.

If you can avoid working a night shift, do so by whatever means possible! Working through the night on a regular basis has been linked to sleep problems, anger, depression and anxiety. This is why many professions that require a night shift typically rotate this shift around so that the employee will only have to work this shift for a month or two at a time, with a few months break in between to allow the body to readjust. Try to maintain a daytime work schedule as much as possible, and if you can control how often you work a night shift, do so as little as possible.

Taking Sleep Seriously

Even the most health conscious, physically fit person will suffer ill consequences if he does not get enough quality sleep. The importance of good sleep to overall health is critical, and its effect on testosterone levels cannot be overstated! While one night of bad sleep here and there may not take you too far off track, several nights of disrupted sleep certainly will. So if this is a pattern for you, it's worth the extra effort to get your sleep cycle on track.

Even if you've never slept longer than five hours a night, try making some adjustments to your light exposure and environment to see if you can maximize your sleep time. Ideally, the best hours to sleep are between the hours of 10pm and 6am, in total darkness and quiet during those hours. With some effort, you may be able to "rewire" your brain and bring your circadian clock back into balance.

Eliminating micro nutrient deficiencies is the easiest way to tackle low testosterone. An estimated 50% of Americans suffer from micro nutrient vitamin deficiencies. If you want to build muscle mass and experience the gains you desire, you must make some lifestyle changes, as well as get the micro nutrients and testosterone to fuel you. Building your body is easy when you have proper testosterone support.

Accelerated aging is growing due to environmental toxins, faster lifestyles, stress and work environments that lock people inside away from the sun and magnify stress levels. The result is fatigue, reduced muscle mass and often depression. This is often tied to low testosterone. The good news is that with lifestyle changes and proper supplementation, the effects can be reversed.

The goal is restoring and balancing testosterone levels without hormone replacements for an all-natural and pure performance boost.

Many men are turning to Human Growth Hormone (HGH) supplementation, but it is wise to tackle lifestyle and nutritional issues before choosing this path. Often people choose HGH therapy prematurely because they have failed to address micro nutrient deficiencies and lifestyle factors. While HGH supplementation does work, if you do not address nutrient deficiencies you will likely need to increase HGH dosages over time, which will eventually inhibit your natural hormone production and ultimately cause the body to stop producing HGH altogether.

The goal is to kick start your own body's natural ability. With our testosterone boosting supplement, for example, we take a straight forward approach and tackle one of the most common health problems, which is nutrient deficiency, while also providing power packed natural ingredients that support testosterone production.

15 VITAMINS, MINERALS AND NATURAL INGREDIENTS THAT BOOST TESTOSTERONE

B VITAMINS

Vitamin B complex (which consists of 8 different water-soluble vitamins, specifically Vitamin B3, Vitamin B6, Vitamin B12, Vitamin B5), is a major player in testosterone production and boosting energy. Deficiency in many B vitamins results in increased estrogen levels, increased prolactin levels, and lowered testosterone levels.

Normally, both men and women have small amounts of prolactin in their blood. Prolactin is a hormone produced by the pituitary gland, which sits at the bottom of the brain. In men, high prolactin levels (hyperprolactinemia) can cause galactorrhea (production of breast milk in men or women who are not breastfeeding), impotence (inability to have an erection during sex), reduced libido (desire for sex), and infertility. A man with untreated hyperprolactinemia may make less sperm, or no sperm at all.

During a woman's pregnancy, prolactin levels go up. Once the baby is born, estrogen and progesterone levels suddenly drop, but high prolactin levels trigger the body to make milk for breastfeeding. In women who aren't pregnant, prolactin helps regulate the menstrual cycle (periods).

For men, however, high prolactin levels in men is not good. To keep it simple, men want *high testosterone*, *low estrogen* and *low prolactin* levels.

In both men's and women's brains, the neurotransmitter that triggers sexuality is acetylcholine (ACH). With too little ACH, sexual activity goes down. A daily dose of a vitamin B complex has been shown to boost ACH, and, as demonstrated above, regulates estrogen, prolactin and testosterone levels.

VITAMIN D

A study by Department of Internal Medicine, Division of Endocrinology and Metabolism, Medical University of Graz, Austria found that supplementation with a dose of 3332 IU's of vitamin D for one full year leads to 25% higher testosterone levels in healthy male subjects. (http://www.ncbi.nlm.nih.gov/pubmed/21154195)

As many as 3/4 of U.S. teens and adults are deficient in vitamin D, and these deficits may contribute to a wide range of health problems, including cancer, heart disease, diabetes - and erectile dysfunction! This deficiency is in large part due to the use of sun screens (which block vitamin D production) and a decrease in outdoor activities. The elderly and those with darker skin are at higher risk for vitamin D deficiency. Sun exposure is a great way to optimize your vitamin D levels, and vitamin D-rich foods and supplements may also be necessary if you cannot get adequate sun exposure year-round.

When it comes to supplements, vitamin D2 is the synthetic form of vitamin D, whereas D3 is the natural form of vitamin D created in your body when you expose your skin to sunlight. D3 produces 2 to 3 times more vitamin D storage in your body than D2, and it converts to the more active form in your body 500 times faster than D2.

ZINC

Zinc plays an essential role in many bodily functions, helping to produce at least 300 enzymes, DNA and repairing cells. Zinc can help you sleep better at night, helps maintain prostate health, and proper levels of zinc also protect against hair loss.

Zinc significantly helps testosterone production, and a deficiency will damage the endocrine system. Zinc might be one of the most important micronutrients for healthy testosterone production. It has been shown to increase testosterone levels in athletes and exercising 'normal' men.

MAGNESIUM

An estimated 80% of Americans are deficient in magnesium. Magnesium helps activate muscles and nerves, creates energy, and helps digest foods. Magnesium is very similar to zinc when it comes to increasing testosterone levels. Deficiency in both will seriously lower testosterone levels, but if your levels of both are already adequate, then additional doses will not do much to help.

Research suggests that most people probably need more magnesium, but you should get blood work by your doctor first to be sure. Magnesium evaporates from the body through sweat, so if you work out daily, or live in a warm and humid environment, then you're probably not getting enough magnesium.

A study done by Karaman High Medicine of Physical Education

and Sports, Selcuk University, in Karaman, Turkey showed showed that supplementation with magnesium increases free and total testosterone values in sedentary individuals and in athletes, with higher increases in those who exercise than in sedentary individuals.

BORON
Boron is a mineral found in food that is important for a variety of body functions, such as regulation of hormones, keeping bones healthy, reducing symptoms of menopause and increasing testosterone. The Sport Physiology Research Center in Baqiyatallah, at University of Medical Sciences, found that subjects consuming a capsule of 10mg boron every day with their breakfast after one week showed significant increases in testosterone.

ASHWAGANDHA
Ashwaganandha is on Dr. Mercola's list of top Adaptogen herbs. Adaptogens are agents that help your body resist occasional stress, anxious feelings, and fatigue. And because they're herbs, they work on your entire body, not just a single area.

Even though the concept of adaptogens dates back thousands of years, modern research didn't begin until the late 1940s. Following World War II, Soviet scientists set out to determine why Siberians lived healthy and long lives – many living beyond 100 years.

Over a period of 45 years, 1200 research scientists conducted over 3,000 studies involving more than 500,000 people. This led to the discovery of "adaptogens," a phrase coined by Dr. Nicolai Lazarev. Together with Dr. Lazarev, Professor Israel Brekhman, the three researched and showed that a new class of plant compounds could help people neutralize stress and live healthier lives.

For an herb to be considered an adaptogen, Professor Brekhman determined that it must:
- Be entirely non-toxic

- Have a "non-specific" activity, increasing the resistance of your entire body rather than any specific organ

- Work to help your entire system gain balance, also called homeostasis

The scientists also felt adaptogens improved the functioning of the entire person by:

- Boosting energy levels and helping enhance longevity
- Promoting good reproductive system health
- Supporting the brain and other essential organs
- Promoting a healthy digestive system
- Helping enhance skeletal and muscular systems

Ashwagandha is a small evergreen perennial herb that grows up to 1.5 meters (almost 5 feet) tall. Common names used for ashwagandha include: Winter Cherry, Withania somnifera (Latin botanical name), and Indian Ginseng, to name a few. Its potential benefits are:

- Boosting endurance, stamina, and sexual energy
- Helping enhance resistance to occasional stress
- Assisting in refreshing both mind and body
- Helping calm and soothe the nervous system
- Aiding in falling asleep naturally

Another interesting factor that separates ashwagandha from some other adaptogens is its effect on the body. While some adaptogens are stimulants in disguise, this is not the case with ashwagandha. It may boost a person's energy or assist in falling asleep, depending on when it is taken in accordance with the body's own circadian rhythm.

CHOLINE

A key nutrient for the human diet is choline. Choline is commonly grouped in the B vitamin family, and it is a key nutrient for the human diet. It is important for many key functions of the body, assisting the brain, liver, cellular, and endocrine system. Choline has also been known to help reduce symptoms of depression, memory loss, and seizures. Endurance athletes also use choline as an aid to build and maintain muscle, as well as combat fatigue throughout peak training periods.

Side effects of low levels of choline include difficulty focusing, low levels of energy, and brain fog. Deficiency can lead to increased threat of a condition known as "Fatty Liver," which results from slowed metabolizing of fat and increased accumulation of lipids in the liver.

Choline deficiency also slows the processes of the nervous system, decreasing vital neurotransmission throughout the body. If the brain does not get enough choline to maintain proper neurotransmission, it may resort to feeding off of cell walls in order to obtain additional choline, leading to a higher risk of memory loss and mental disorders.

Once your body receives a dose of choline, it provokes neurotransmitters that prompt the release of nitric oxide, which is said to be the main chemical mediator of erectile functioning. Essentially, choline sets off the chain reaction that results in a healthy erection.

Choline may also improve mood, energy, and motivation, which all contribute to a healthy sex drive.

EURYCOMA LONGIFOLIA (TONGKAT ALI)
Tongkat Ali is a flowering plant native to Indonesia, Malaysia.

The active ingredients claimed to increase testosterone include steroidal saponins and eurycomanone. There's also some aphrodisiac pro-erectile compounds in the herb, such as Canthin-6-one metabolites and derivatives of Squalene.

If you've done any amount of research about boosting testosterone, most likely you've already come across Tongkat Ali.

In a 6+ month long study conducted by the School of Medical Sciences at the Universiti Sains Malaysia, researchers conducted a double blind study of 109 participants. They gave half of these men 300 mg's of freeze dried Tongkat Ali extract, and the other half got placebo. After 12 weeks, the participants in the Tongkat Ali group showed significant increases in semen motility and volume, as well as improved erectile function and libido. (http://www.ncbi.nlm.nih.gov/pubmed/23243445)

PHOSPHATIDYLSERINE
You read about PS in chapter 1, but it is definitely among the most important testosterone boosting agents, so it's worth noting again here. Eat plenty of pastured meats, white beans and tuna, or

be sure your daily supplement contains a healthy dose of PS.

L-ARGININE

According to Dr. Joseph Mercola:

As far as natural alternatives go, there are many options to consider, including L-arginine, an amino acid that is the precursor to nitric oxide, a natural compound that helps relax your blood vessels. Nitric oxide signals the smooth muscle cells in your blood vessels to relax, so that your vessels dilate and your blood flows more freely. This helps your arteries to regain their elasticity and stay free of plaque. L-arginine may also lead to increased microcirculation in genital tissues, which results in stronger erections and better sexual responsiveness, via this nitric oxide mechanism.

In fact, this is how a leading ED drug treats erectile problems — it increases nitric oxide production, relaxing your blood vessels, which increases penile blood flow. However, the price you might pay for these ED drugs is a slew of potentially dangerous side effects, including reducing blood pressure too low. L-arginine increases the action of nitric oxide — similar to ED drugs, but without the side effects.

Scientific studies have shown that L-arginine can be particularly effective when used in combination with another natural agent, pycnogenol, which resulted in significant improvement in sexual function in men with ED, according to a Bulgarian study.8 Similarly, a pilot study published in the journal European Urology found six grams of L-arginine combined with six mg of yohimbine, a compound found in the herb yohimbe, was successful in treating men with ED

8 source http://www.ncbi.nlm.nih.gov/pubmed/12851125
9 source http://www.ncbi.nlm.nih.gov/pubmed/12074777

HORNY GOAT WEED

Horny goat weed (Epimedium) is a flowering plant, native to the Mediterranean region of Asia. For centuries, it has been used as a powerful aphrodisiac in Chinese medicine. It contains high levels of the compound called icariin, which is reputed through many in-vitro and animal studies for boosting testosterone levels.

Some of the studies revealed that icariin can suppress the stress hormone cortisol. And as you've read in earlier chapters, keeping cortisol in check is hugely important to boosting testosterone levels.

Can Women Benefit From Boosting Testosterone?

Although we often think in the simplistic terms of testosterone for men, estrogen for women, testosterone also plays an important role in women's biology.

Many women have a difficulty maintaining their sex drive after menopause, which could be the result of lowering testosterone levels. Some studies have shown that testosterone patches have helped revive that sex drive, revealing that efforts to naturally boost testosterone may be helpful for menopausal women, as well.

Testosterone also helps women keep bones healthy. Maintaining a proper level of testosterone will support the growth and strength of healthy bones, whereas too little can potentially contribute to osteoporosis.

Testosterone contributes to overall muscle tone, and since pelvic muscles are particularly dependent on testosterone, boosting testosterone levels in women can help them overcome leaky bladder issues.

But testosterone is not just for menopausal women. Just as in men, testosterone can help women increase muscle tone and burn fat more efficiently. Weight lifting increases testosterone in women, and in fact women who lift weights and work out with their husband report having improved sex lives. Women who are deficient in testosterone report that feelings of improved overall wellbeing after taking measures to boost their T-levels.

For women who have had their ovaries removed, testosterone may drop by up to 50 percent. They often report that they do not feel the same, are not as strong, and lack energy and sex drive. Additionally, women who are undergoing hormone replacement therapy will need to take measures to boost their testosterone, as increased estrogen levels can reduce testosterone production.

One of the most favorable reported effects testosterone boosting efforts has on women is how it performs as a powerful anti-aging agent. Women produce increased amounts of testosterone during puberty, and their levels peak in their early 20's. Women who use oral contraceptives often suffer a decline in testosterone, as birth control pills suppress all hormone production. By the time a woman reaches menopause, she may have less than half of the testosterone she had in her youth.

Efforts for boosting testosterone can greatly benefit women, just as it can for men. Proper testosterone levels in women burn fat into muscle, increase skin elasticity and bone density, improve mood, increase the ability to handle stress, and increase sexual drive. There is also evidence that shows proper levels of testosterone in women can support brain function, as well as maintain clean liver and blood vessels.

SUPER MALE OPTIMIZER

Our unique blend of micronutrients and powerful herbs sets our formula apart from other testosterone boosters on the market today. If your body is deficient in key vitamins and nutrients, it simply will not respond efficiently to any other efforts to boost your testosterone, improve performance or optimize your health. The bonus is that these nutrients help protect your health, while also supporting increased testosterone levels.

Additionally, when it comes to taking vitamins, absorption is key. Why waste money on expensive supplements if your body does not absorb them? SUPER MALE OPTIMIZER contains high quality, and highly absorbable vitamins, minerals, amino acids and herbs.

We've paid attention to what you need to achieve optimal health and wellness, and then we add the most potent ingredients known for boosting testosterone levels. Our multivitamin + T-booster is built to the highest standards, is non-GMO, and every batch is third party tested to guarantee quality. Click here to get your bottle of our natural testosterone booster today!

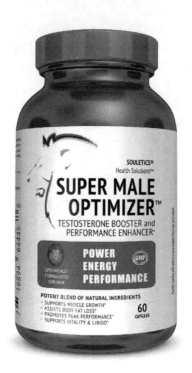

CHAPTER 4: Gut Health and Probiotics

Chances are by now you've heard some talk about the connection between your gut and your overall health, and about the importance of taking probiotics on a daily basis. But did you know that the human body is actually made up of over 100 trillion bacterial cells, as opposed to only 10 trillion human cells? From a cellular perspective, we are only 10% human!

Only recently is the medical community coming to grips with what a big deal this is. In 2008, the National Institute of Health launched the Human Microbiome Project, an effort to identify the microbiology of both healthy and diseased humans in five distinct body sites: the gut, mouth, nose/lung, vagina and skin. Much more recently, in May of 2016, the White House announced a half-billion-dollar project to study the communities of microbes that colonize almost everything on Earth, from animals, to soil, the ocean, and the atmosphere.

This immense population of microbes that inhabits our bodies and environment is often referred to as the "microbiome," and it is somewhat like finding an entirely new planet contained right here on Earth. And like any living ecosystem, there are the good guys and the bad guys, and if the bad guys start to outnumber the good guys, you're bound to see trouble on the horizon.

That's the simple way to look at probiotics – they're the good guys. And there are a wide range of types, or "strains," of these good guys who act like special forces against the pathogens, fungi and parasites whose goal it is to intercept the nutrients you ingest. These bad guys also crave junk food, so if you find yourself with junk food cravings, most likely your microbiome is out of whack. So you want to enlist as many specialists as possible to fight off the invaders and other organisms that have likely taken over the neighborhood in your gut.

Benefits of Taking Probiotics

In general, probiotics can increase your overall well being simply by keeping your microbiome in balance. They can improve how your digestive system functions and boost your immune system. But there are a number of specific ailments probiotics have also been proven to treat, including:

- Urinary tract infections
- Inflammatory bowel conditions like IBS
- Eczema
- Food borne illness

More recent studies are beginning to reveal advances in probiotics against these conditions, as well:
- Flu and colds
- Kidney stones
- Colic
- Cavities and gum disease
- Colitis and Crohn's disease
- Liver disease
- Cancer
- Autism
- Ulcers
- Acne
- Weight gain

Unfortunately, probiotics are transient, meaning they do not implant themselves in your system the way the pathogens, fungi, viruses and other bad bacteria do when they've outnumbered the good guys. Your body can reestablish its own natural beneficial bacteria, but it takes time and a concerted effort to keep your system clear of pathogens while healing your digestive tract from any damage the offenders may have caused. The good news is that there is a protocol for doing this; it's called the "GAPS Diet" (based on the book *Gut And Psychology Syndrome* by Dr. Natasha Campbell-McBride), and it is designed to heal a variety of ailments simply by healing your digestive system. If you're interested, we'll have more information on that in the next chapter.

How to Take Probiotics: Managing Side Effects
If you've never taken a probiotic, you may experience "side effects" when you begin a probiotic treatment. These side effects are unlike the conditions we're accustomed to hearing about at the end of most commercials for pharmaceutical drugs; they are not long lasting, do not damage other organs or cause unheard of

diseases, and rarely do they cause negative interactions with other drugs or foods you may consume. However, during the first few days when you begin taking probiotics for the first time you may actually feel as though you're coming down with the flu. You may be foggy headed, have headaches, feel nauseous, experience diarrhea or bloating, get the chills, and any symptoms that caused you to take the probiotic in the first place (i.e. skin rashes, yeast infection, digestive issues, etc) may actually flare up even worse than before. This is called the "Herxheimer Reaction," and it occurs when the microorganisms within your body release endotoxins as they begin to die off. The most common offender is candida (yeast), but it could be any other bacteria, virus or pathogens that have also taken hold in your body.

This is not uncommon when you start a detox regime; most often you'll feel much worse before you begin to feel better. For this reason, however, it's a good idea to start with a small army (i.e. a milder probiotic with fewer strains and only a few billion live cultures per capsule) and work your way up to the special forces (i.e. a stronger dosage with more strains and hundreds of billions of live cultures per capsule). Otherwise it may feel as though a bomb went off in your stomach and you'll be miserable for days, even weeks, on end.

If this happens, and especially if it comes on hard, back off the probiotic to about half of the dose you took in the first place, and then work your way up a little more each day until the symptoms subside. It's actually a good sign, it just means those bad guys are dying off faster than your body can remove them and the substances they release as they say their final farewell.

For example, when yeast cells are rapidly killed, they actually release 79 different toxins, including ethanol and acetaldehyde. These toxins are extremely detrimental to your health, so it's important to make sure you're doing all you can to flush these chemicals from your system.

It's important to drink plenty of water, and if your symptoms are strong or last longer than a day or two, it would be a good idea to incorporate a milk thistle supplement or drink dandelion tea to support your liver as it's deluged with this influx of toxins. As much as you may want to work out and sweat it out, it's a better idea to get as much rest as possible and let your body heal itself. A warm bath in Epsom salt or a hot sauna followed by a cold shower may help.

Once your symptoms have subsided and you begin to feel better, you should notice your bowel movements occurring on a more regular schedule. If not, increase your dosage little by little until you experience regularity.

How Probiotics Impact Testosterone Production

In addition to the plethora of benefits probiotics have to offer the rest of your body, they have also been shown to boost testosterone production in men. This happens through a number of mechanisms, mainly by lowering the stress hormone cortisol, which, as you have read previously, inhibits testosterone production. But another study in particular showed that regular doses of probiotics may also have the following direct impact on men:

- prevent age related testicular shrinkage
- increase testicular size and weight
- increase testosterone levels significantly
- increase activity of hypothalamus-pituitary-testis axis
- increase sperm motility, quality and quantity
- increase luteinizing hormone and follicle stimulating hormone levels

What type of probiotic is most effective?

So does this mean you should start eating more yogurt? Not if that yogurt bears a commercial name and is loaded with sugar. Most of the yogurts you find in your grocery store are no better for you than ice cream, and if they ever had a live culture in the first place, by the time they reach your mouth the chances are good that they're dead.

Don't get me wrong – yogurt is a very healthy food to consume on a regular basis, and a high quality yogurt can provide your body with some beneficial bacteria. But the best quality will be the kind you make at home (it's really not difficult, and we have a very simple recipe for you to follow in the next chapter), and even then, it should not be your only source of probiotics.

The best approach to probiotics is a varied one. As stated above, once you begin working your way up to higher doses of probiotics, you want to enlist as many specialists as possible. This means incorporating a high quality probiotic supplement in addition to consuming fermented foods. There are some strains of probiotics found in fermented foods that simply won't be found in a probiotic supplement. But fermented foods on their own just won't provide the quantity of troops that you need to chase out the foreign invaders.

It also goes without saying that you'll also want to begin eliminating the types of foods that feed the foreign troops. Your goal is to create as hostile an environment for those guys as possible, so you certainly don't want to continue giving them the foods they crave. On the contrary, you want to consume the types of foods that nourish the good guys, because that's the exact food that will nourish you, as well.

So keep reading, because in the following chapters we'll provide shopping tips, recipes, and foods you can enjoy when eating out that will restore balance in your gut and ultimately BOOST your TESTOSTERONE!

ULTIMATE GUT HEALTH

Our probiotic "Ultimate Gut Health" contains seven of the most important strains of beneficial bacteria: Bifidobacterium Longum, Lactobacillus Rhamnosus, Lactobacillus Casei, Lactobacillus Acidophilus, Lactobacillus Plantarum, Lactobacilluls Breve, and Bacillus Subtilis.

The perfect companion to SUPER MALE OPTIMIZER, both are now available on Amazon.com. Click here to purchase our gentle and effective blend of high quality probiotic!

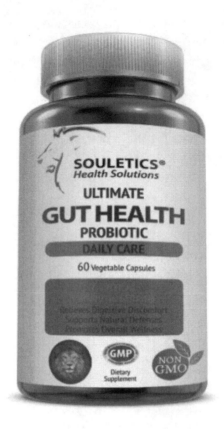

As mentioned in the previous chapter, the GAPS diet is an effective protocol for healing the gut, as well as restoring your digestive and immune system. Though it was written with a primary focus of treating patients diagnosed with autism, the diet has been widely reported to help people heal from a variety of ailments, including:

* Acne
* A.D.D. & A.D.H.D.
* Asthma and Seasonal Allergies
* Auto-immune diseases, such as Multiple Sclerosis, Fibromyalgia, Chronic Fatigue Syndrome, etc.
* Bipolar Disorder
* Depression
* Dermatitis, Eczema, Psoriasis
* Food Intolerances
* Irritable Bowel Syndrome
* Krohn's Disease
* Schizophrenia

It is not a fad diet, but it shares some similarities with the trendy paleo diet – mainly in the avoidance of grains, sugars and dairy (except fermented and raw dairy for those who can tolerate it), while integrating traditional fermented foods and broth for healing the gut. While a true GAPS diet is more involved than what I will share in this book, I've incorporated some of its basic rules and ways to convert recipes to meet GAPS standards. If you are suffering from any of the above ailments, however, I highly encourage you to do your research on GAPS and see if it's a right fit for you.

The Basic Food Rules for Restoring Your Gut

The bad news is that, depending on your starting point, you may need to weed out old favorites from your diet. But the great news is that when you eat the right foods that keep your gut in balance, you don't have to obsess about cutting calories or starving yourself. In fact, by making these dietary adjustments, you should feel much more satiated without that overly stuffed and heavy feeling.

1. **Fill your diet with as many whole foods as possible** – the kind that don't come in a box or package. Apples, bananas, carrots, avocados, celery, cheese, nuts, nut butter... we'll have a list of healthy fast foods in the next section.

2. **No processed junk food.** That includes candy bars, boxed meal starters, chips, crisps, soda, energy drinks, boxed cereals, cookies, even so called "healthy" granola bars that are loaded with sugar and grains. Read the label. If you see high fructose corn syrup, colors followed by numbers, or any ingredients you can't pronounce, leave it alone!

3. **No fast food.** Period. Exclamation point! We'll go over some healthy alternatives in the next section.

4. **Keep sugar and grains to a minimum.** Again, read food labels! Feed any cravings for sweets with raw unrefined honey, nut butters, fruits and dried fruits. Grains are especially important to avoid if you're having health issues, but even if you're not, do your best to keep grain based foods (especially wheat flour) in the minority of foods you eat.

5. **Drink plenty of water.** Aim for drinking half your body weight in ounces each day of pure, clean water. Get a good filter and reusable water bottle to minimize the amount of plastics you consume.

6. **No sodas, and no fruit juice.** Almost all pre-packaged fruit juices (even the organic ones) have been pasteurized and rid of all beneficial nutrients. By the time they've been bottled, contained in a warehouse, distributed for miles, and transported to your mouth, they're not all that much different than a can of soda, as far as the sugar content is concerned. There may be some remnant of a vitamin contained in the juice, but it's just not worth the influx of sugar to your system.

7. **Opt for fresh, cold pressed juice.** Fresh, cold pressed juices are a great alternative to bottled fruit juice, and there are plenty of juiceries cropping up now that juice cleanses are becoming more popular. This is a good, albeit expensive, habit to get into, but if you find yourself getting hooked, invest in a juicer of your own and play around with the flavors you enjoy. Try to stick with at least half vegetable based juice and half fruit based juice for optimum nutritional results.

8. **Stay away from vegetable oil, including canola oil.** These oils are cheap, processed with dangerous chemicals, and they become highly unstable when exposed to heat. They're also extremely high in Omega 6 fats. The best oils to cook with, which remain stable at high temperatures, include coconut oil (refined for frying, unrefined for eating and baking), avocado oil, ghee, and grass fed lard (no, lard is not bad for you if it comes from a good source!). The best oils to use in salad dressings and non-cooked foods include cold pressed olive oils, avocado oil, flaxseed oil, walnut oil, and macadamia nut oil. Sesame and peanut oils are also good for use in moderation.

9. **Buy organic as much as possible.** Foods that have not been treated with pesticides not only are free from the toxic load of those poisons, but numerous recent studies have revealed that organic foods have more antioxidants and micronutrients than conventional foods. One theory states that organic plants develop chemicals to protect themselves from pathogens, and when we consume those plants we reap the benefit of those chemicals fighting off pathogens in our bodies, as well. These pathogen fighting substances are not found in conventional plants that rely on pesticides to do the work for them. Regardless of "why" organic plants have more cancer fighting compounds like antioxidants and polyphenols, the research shows they are far superior to conventional foods, so do your best to always buy organic; or better yet, try to do your main shopping at a farmers market near you!

10. **Know the "dirty dozen."** These are the most contaminated fruits and veggies, and they include peaches, apples, bell peppers, celery, nectarines, strawberries, cherries, pears, grapes, spinach, lettuce and potatoes. If you can't afford organic across the board, strive to buy these organic, and as many other thin-skinned or root based produce, since they have little protection from the pesticides in the soil. Produce with a thicker skin (bananas, citrus) or any produce you can peel can be relegated to conventional until you can afford to do better!

11. **Cook as much as you possibly can from scratch**. If you're not into spending time in the kitchen, this rule may seem excessively harsh. However, when you learn a few basic techniques, you'll quickly realize this isn't nearly as difficult as it seems. And this one rule alone can help you refrain from over indulging. Can you eat fried chicken wings and pizza for dinner with root beer and ice cream for dessert? If your rule is to make it from scratch, using whole, fresh, organic ingredients, you'd be prepping this meal for days before you can actually enjoy it. But you can develop a repertoire of simple, fresh recipes that are delicious and easy to make from scratch. Over time you'll learn to think and prep ahead and you'll develop the skills to make more indulgent foods that won't throw your diet (and gut) off balance.

12. **Choose bread selectively and eat it in moderation.** Even though wheat is not technically a GMO, it has been adulterated for generations, probably more than any other American crop, and non-organic wheat is heavily sprayed with loads of toxic pesticides. On top of that, refined flour essentially turns into sugar in your body, spiking your insulin levels and creating inflammation. Even when you think you're eating something healthy by choosing "whole grain" bread, most likely your body is not reaping the benefit because grains actually contain "anti-nutrients" that keep your body from digesting them and reaping the benefits of those nutrients. The best bread that can be easily digested and is full of vitamins, minerals, antioxidants, and even

protein, is made with sprouted or fermented (i.e. sourdough) grains. Fortunately, now those aren't too difficult to find, but just make sure to read the labels and make sure the grains are organic and not mixed with heavy amounts of refined flour or sugar. If you choose sourdough, make sure you buy one that's traditionally fermented and not made with quick-starters that mimic the flavor of sourdough while bypassing the healthy fermenting process. If you're gluten intolerant, be cautious about the gluten free breads you buy, as most rely on starches and sugars to compensate for the missing gluten ingredient. The gluten free varieties that incorporate "ancient grains," millet, buckwheat and chia are the best bet.

13. **Throw away your boxed cereals, even the organic ones.** If you've been known to stock up on breakfast cereals and consuming them whenever you want a crunchy sweet fix, this is one habit you'll want to ditch fast. Cereal does nothing for your body nutritionally, and the way the grains are processed into puffs, crisps, shreds and shapes is by a method called "extrusion," which is actually quite toxic. The Weston A. Price Foundation published a very in-depth look at the cereal industry on their website called "Dirty Secrets of the Food Processing Industry," and well worth the read if you're having any trouble getting past your cereal addiction (visit www.westonaprice.org or search "cereal WAPF" to locate the article). For a decent replacement, we've got an easy granola recipe in the next chapter.

And now for the good stuff...

What to Eat to Boost Testosterone Levels
1. **Fat.** Yes, you read that right. Fat. You may have been expecting recipes involving lean, white chicken breasts, but you won't find those here. Studies show that diets incorporating 40% of calories from high quality fat show higher testosterone levels than diets with 25% or less of calories from fat. It turns out that after years of villainizing fat and cholesterol for causing heart disease, the docs had it wrong all along – it's the low quality fats and processed,

refined grains causing all the heartache. The catch is that in order to reap the benefits of fat, it must come from high quality, pastured animals and organic fruits, vegetables and nuts, and you must avoid refined sugars and carbohydrates. Otherwise, the combination of fat, sugar and carbs will only lead you back down the road to an imbalanced gut and low testosterone.

2. **In particular, consume healthy Omega 3 fat.** To get specific, the research points to the imbalance of Omega 3 to Omega 6 in Western diets as the main culprit for our epidemic of chronic illness. This imbalance creates inflammation that can quickly snowball into any variety of disease. Omega 3 fats decrease inflammation and are the most important fats to consume, but we need both in our diet; we just need them in proper balance. Since Omega 6 fats are less expensive, the Standard American Diet (SAD) is heavy on the Omega 6 side. Where most nutritionists agree the optimal ratio is 1:1, the SAD Western Diet has an imbalanced ratio of 15 (Omega 6) to 1 (Omega 3)!! The best thing you can do is eat as many foods that are rich in Omega 3, and try to limit the foods high in Omega 6. The more Omega 3 fats you consume, the less Omega 6 will be available in your body to create inflammation. So more Omega 3 = less inflammation. **Foods high in Omega 3 include: fatty fish (mackerel, salmon, cod, tuna, herring), walnuts, chia seeds, flax seeds, hemp seeds, anchovies, egg yolks, and grass fed beef.** The foods highest in Omega 6 (foods you should avoid) include vegetable oil, commercial salad dressings & mayonnaise, nuts & seeds (these are still good to eat, just don't overdo it), processed snack foods, commercial pork sausages, commercial chicken and feed-lot beef. This is also why it's best to eat pastured meats – because commercially raised livestock and poultry are fed cheap feed that is high in Omega 6, whereas pastured animals eat the way nature intended, which is high in Omega 3 fats.

3. **Bone broth.** Due in large part to the GAPS diet, broth has made a huge splash among health food enthusiasts. An

integral part of Eastern traditional foods and Chinese medicine for hundreds of years, broth is known for healing the digestive tract and providing plenty of minerals and nutrients that support various other functions of the body. It turns out that it also helps boost testosterone via a relatively recently discovered protein known as osteocalcin, which is produced by bone cells. It acts as a hormone and regulates numerous bodily functions, including signaling the testes to make more testosterone!

4. **Consume plenty of fermented foods.** Not only will fermented foods help keep your gut in balance, but sauerkraut and kefir are great sources of vitamin K2, which is known for increasing testosterone levels. Kefir also provides your body with healthy levels zinc, another testosterone booster and prostate protector. Kefir is one of the easiest fermented foods to make, and you'll find instructions for making it (and recipes for using it) in the next chapter.

5. **Eat raw honey.** As mentioned above, sugar consumption should be kept to a minimum. Raw, unfiltered honey, however, is your friend! Most commercial honey is very low quality and just as bad as eating sugar, but if you get a locally sourced raw honey, it will contain healing compounds – including boron and chrysin, minerals that reduce the conversion of testosterone into estrogen, and nitric oxide, which has been found to strengthen erections by opening blood vessels. Legend has it, this is where the term "honeymoon" originated.

6. **Load up on garlic and onions.** Studies involving rats showed that garlic supplementation increased testicular testosterone while decreasing cortisol. Animals fed with onion juice showed similar gains, as well as increased sperm quality.

7. **Cold pressed extra virgin olive oil.** A study on olive oil among healthy adult Moroccan men showed significant increases of T levels after only 3 weeks of supplementing extra virgin olive oil in these men's diet.

8. **Blueberries, Pineapple, Bananas, Pomegranate and Ginger.**
    Sounds like the makings of a tasty smoothie, but each are
    great sources for supporting high testosterone levels.
    Blueberries are high in Resveratrol, which controls estrogen
    levels, and Calcium-D-Glucarate, which increases natural T
    production. Bananas and pineapple are high in the enzyme
    Bromelain, which is a widely reported T booster. Studies
    involving ginger showed that it can actually boost T levels in
    infertile men. And pomegranate has been shown to boost
    nitric oxide, which, as indicated above, strengthens
    erections. However, another study indicated that daily doses
    of pomegranate may increase T levels by up to 21%.

Healthy Fast Foods

It takes a bit of planning and preparation to maintain a clean
eating regime, but it's well worth the effort. Get in the habit of
stocking up weekly and taking a day or two during the week to prep
foods for busy days or long outings.

Here are some good snacks to prep and have on hand for busy
days. If you take one day to slice, dice and separate into
containers, you can grab and go and save yourself from the
temptations of vending machines and unhealthy fast food.

- Carrot sticks

- Celery & nut butter or cheese

- Apples, bananas, seasonal fruit

- Avocados

- Cucumbers, olives & Greek yogurt

- Hard boiled pastured eggs

- Good quality (nitrate free/organic) lunch meat & cheese

- "Bubbies" dill pickles (traditionally fermented pickles with
  live probiotic cultures, the Bubbies brand is probably the
  best quality, and possibly even the only fermented pickle,
  you can find in most grocery stores)

- Nuts, dried fruit & homemade trail mix

- Plain yogurt with fruit & honey

- Salads (recipes in the next chapter)

Healthy Alternatives When Eating Out

Eating out regularly is a sure way to ruin your testosterone boosting food regime. Unless you're surrounded by 5-star farm-to-fork restaurants and wealthy enough to foot that fine dining bill, it's simply not possible to maintain a budget friendly clean diet if you're frequenting restaurants.

However, sometimes you can't avoid eating out. Work demands, social events, and other situations sometimes make it tough to get a home cooked meal. So in the rare instances when you have to eat out, here are some ways to enjoy the experience without wreaking havoc on your gut.

- Think protein and vegetables. And no, French fries do not count as vegetables. You want colorful veggies and beans, legumes, or meats.

- Soup could be a good option, but try to avoid creamy, cheesy or pasta filled varieties.

- No fried foods. Not just because they're fried, but because they're fried in cheap oil that turns completely toxic when heated.

- Avoid bread and sweets.

- If you have the option to choose where you eat, go for the place that has the freshest food possible (preferably not the type of restaurant that features a drive thru) in whole form. A local ethnic restaurant is probably your best bet, as many still utilize fresh foods and traditional cooking methods, or even a Chipotle grill if there is nothing better available.

- If you wind up at a burger joint, request your burger wrapped in lettuce instead of a bun (and make sure you get a fork and knife to avoid the mess). Standard non-organic veggie burgers are often loaded with inflammatory carbs, pesticides and other unhealthy ingredients, so you're probably best off with a bun-less carnivorous option. However, some restaurants make their own veggie, bean or nut burgers that could be worth a try.

- If you're on the road traveling and just need a pit stop for lunch or snacks, try to find a grocery store – especially one with a decent deli and fresh soup or salads – or any place you can buy something fresh. Some coffee shops now sell protein plates with a hard boiled egg, cheese, fruit and nuts. Juice and smoothie shops are also a good bet, but be careful to avoid sugary processed juices and smoothies made with sherbet or other refined ingredients.

- If your travel route only offers you convenience stores, stick with nuts and water. Beef jerky is also an option, but most commercial brands are high in sugar and nitrates, so unless you luck up on a locally sourced or higher quality brand, it's best to leave that alone.

- Intermittent fasting is always an option! Aside from the spiritual benefits that fasting brings, studies show that skipping meals on a weekly basis, and even going a day or more at a time without food on a regular basis, is one of the best things you can do for your body and may actually prolong your lifespan. So if you're in a situation where healthy food is unavailable, drink pure clean water and wait it out. Praying and reading scripture can help get you through the hunger waves.

Remember that most restaurants, especially chain restaurants, serve food that is extremely high in sodium and sugar, not to mention a smorgasbord of chemicals, so do your best to keep eating out at a minimum. And when you do eat out, for the rest of the day be sure to drink plenty of water to flush out the bad stuff, and watch what else you eat to minimize the negative effects.

If you're new to cooking, this chapter can help you figure out what to buy so you can prepare your own foods on a daily basis. These are the basic necessities, but of course there's always room to explore and add to your collection as you grow your kitchen skills. Don't worry about breaking the bank to buy everything high end. Probably the most important thing is to try to get stainless steel and/or good old fashioned cast iron, and avoid plastics and chemically treated non-stick cookware. Bamboo spoons and silicon spatulas are relatively inexpensive and safe, and tempered glass casserole dishes will be just fine until your cooking skills warrant the more expensive stoneware or enamel coated cookware.

It is, however, a good idea to invest in tempered glass food containers with lids for storing food, to avoid plastics and aluminum foil, which can also leach chemicals into your food. These are well worth the expense, as they will last you forever and save the toxins, waste and expense that come with unnecessary food packaging.

The list below of tools, gadgets and foods is by no means exhaustive, but it's also not all required at once. Read through the recipes and see what looks good to you, then buy what's required for those recipes.

Once you get in the habit of cooking regularly, you should be able to identify the common ingredients you'll always need to keep on hand in order to make a meal from scratch any day of the week. It helps to make a weekly meal plan and corresponding grocery so that you can buy everything you need in one weekly grocery outing.

Note: I've also created this page on the Souletics Resource Center with links pointing to where you can purchase each item. The page is available at: www.souleticsresourcecenter.com/how-to-stock-your-first-kitchen

Cooking Tools
- Pots and pans: Stainless steel is best, as non-stick cookware is chemically treated and can leach dangerous substances into your food. Try to get 1 large pot, 1 medium pot, 1 large frying pan, 1 small frying pan, and 1 medium sized cast iron skillet.

- Strainers: One for pasta and another fine mesh for straining rice, quinoa and other fine grains
- Dinner plates, salad plates, and soup bowls
- Glasses & mugs
- Large salad bowl
- Large mixing bowl
- Utensils, mixing spoons, spatulas, whisks
- Sharp knives – one serrated, one "French chef" wide blade for cutting vegetables, one butcher knife
- Cutting board: Wood and plastic can harbor bacteria, so a tempered glass cutting board would be best.
- Measuring cups and spoons
- Cheese grater
- Can opener
- Carrot peeler
- Reusable glass or stainless steel water bottle
- Kitchen towels
- Cloth napkins
- Plastic gallon size & sandwich size bags
- Large, Medium & Small food containers

Gadgets:
- Water filter (preferably one that filters out fluoride, like the "Perfect Water Purifier" or a Big Berkey)
- Small Magic Bullet type blender and or more robust "Ninja" style blender
- Slow cooker – VitaClay is our favorite, as it is not chemically treated and won't leach lead or other chemicals into your food. You can also use it to make your own yogurt.
- If you're on GAPS or just into veggie noodles, get a spiralizer!

Pantry

- High quality sea salt (Himalayan or Celtic is best)
- Seasonings: pepper, granulated garlic, spice blend (to your liking – one we like combines garlic, onion, paprika, sea salt and pepper, it tastes great on everything), smoked paprika, cumin, chili pepper, chipotle pepper, cayenne pepper, bay leaves, sage, basil, thyme, oregano, cinnamon, pure vanilla extract, and any other seasonings you like – have fun experimenting!
- Unrefined coconut oil, cold pressed extra virgin olive oil, avocado oil, toasted sesame oil
- Green tea, chai tea (tea bags, not a mix), herbal teas, etc.
- Jarred or canned tuna
- Jarred or canned olives
- Organic canned tomatoes: crushed tomatoes, chopped tomatoes, fire roasted tomatoes, stewed tomatoes with basil and garlic
- Organic canned tomato sauce & tomato paste
- Grass fed Gelatin & Collagen: Grass fed gelatin is a great way to add more protein and gut-healing collagen to your diet. This is where the concept of "Jell-O" came from – can you believe it used to be healthy? Not any more, unless you make your own. Commercial brands are highly processed, adding sugar, artificial colors, and other unhealthy additives that you don't want to consume. But with grass fed gelatin, you can make your own fruit snacks, jell-o, pudding and GAPS legal gravies, and rest assured that they contain some nutritional value. If you're not into the gelatin consistency, you can also buy powdered collagen to add to smoothies and drinks that will add the boost of collagen and protein without altering the consistency at all.
- Safe sweeteners: Raw honey, organic pure maple syrup, coconut palm sugar (unless you're on GAPS, then raw honey is the only GAPS legal sweetener)
- Nut butter: Almond butter is best, preferably sprouted, but that gets expensive! Peanut butter is an inexpensive

alternative, but try to stick with organic and unsweetened (just peanuts and salt in the ingredients)

- Flours: Almond meal, coconut flour, and if you're not on GAPS, cornmeal

- Oats: Organic rolled oats or steel cut

- It's always good to have an organic all purpose flour on hand, preferably a gluten free blend

- Baking powder and baking soda

- If not on GAPS, it's also good to have some form of pasta on hand: brown rice pasta and quinoa pasta are good gluten free varieties, but if you can tolerate wheat it's not a bad idea to have a high quality organic pasta on hand (just be careful not to overcook it)

- Dry navy beans, dry lentils (we like red and black), and if not on GAPS, white basmati rice, dry black, red, pinto and garbanzo beans

- It's also a good idea to have a few cans of beans on hand, for when you don't have the time to soak and cook ahead of time

- Salsa

- High quality organic mayonnaise (for when you don't have time to make your own)

- Nuts, whole food nutrition bars, dried fruit

- Sparkling water

Refrigerator

- Raw, unfiltered apple cider vinegar

- High quality probiotic

- Grass fed/pastured butter: If you're in Northern California, Humboldt Creamery Butter is a great find, but Kerrygold butter is also very good and available in most grocery stores nationwide.

- Eggs: Ideally pastured, but strive to buy the best quality you can afford.

- Bubbies pickles & relish

- Coconut milk

- Plain yogurt

- Cultured sour cream

- Organic/raw milk grass fed cheese: bricks only. Soft cheese molds quickly when shredded, so most bags of pre-shredded cheese require additives to extend the shelf life. If you want shredded cheese, you'll need to use your cheese grater!

- High quality parmesan cheese: Since parmesan is a hard cheese, it can be pre-shredded without requiring additives for preventing mold (although some commercial brands still add them to extend shelf life). So a tub of pre-grated is fine – especially if it was freshly grated by the deli department of a grocery store – but it's still always best to buy a brick and shred or grate your own.

- Lunch meat – nitrate free and organic

Produce

If you're too busy to make it to a farmers market every week, find out if you have a CSA (community supported agriculture) in your area that will make weekly deliveries of farm fresh produce to your doorstep. The one we have (FarmFreshtoYou.com) is very reasonable and even allows you to select what items you want delivered in your box.

Otherwise, try to work into your schedule a weekly visit to the farmers market to make sure you're getting local, fresh fruit and vegetables. It's almost always a better price than what you'll find at grocery stores – healthier food that's locally sourced, and it supports your local farmers.

- Salad greens: Spinach, lettuce, cabbage

- Smoothie greens: Kale, Chard, Collard Greens, Bok Choi

- Fruit: Apples, bananas, lemons, limes, oranges, pineapple, melon... whatever's in season!

- Fresh herbs: Sage, basil, cilantro are our favorites, but have fun experimenting! It's also pretty easy and cost effective to grow herbs in a box in your kitchen window or on your patio.

- Onions, green onions, garlic

- Fresh tomatoes

Freezer

- Frozen veggies are good to have on hand: broccoli, spinach, peas and corn (no corn if on GAPS)

- Frozen fruit can also be good for making smoothies, especially if you like varieties of fruit that don't grow locally, or aren't in season where you live

- If you have a local butcher or grocery store that sells soup bones, stock up in your freezer! Or if you cook meat that has bones but don't have time to immediately make broth, don't throw those bones out – rinse them off and put them in a freezer bag so you can make broth later.

- Safe desserts: Plain frozen yogurt, fruit-only sorbets (make sure there are no added sugars or other off limit ingredients)

Healthy Habits

Every morning, drink a tablespoon of apple cider vinegar, followed by 8-16 ounces of water, along with your probiotic. If you can't stand the taste of vinegar alone, you can dilute it with water, or even add equal parts honey to vinegar, fill it with water and shake it in your shaker jar to blend. It can be an acquired taste, but this is great for your digestive system, and a requirement if you feel a cold coming on. ACV cuts mucous and can shorten the duration of a cold or keep it from developing into something nasty.

Keep your water filter and reusable water bottle filled up, and make sure you're drinking half your body weight in ounces of clean water daily. Staying hydrated will keep you alert and running on all cylinders, and it will also keep you from mistaking dehydration for hunger.

If you like the taste of the unrefined coconut oil, eat 1-2 tablespoons straight each day. This is good for detoxification, so if you feel a little ill after your first few days of trying this out, don't worry – it's your body expelling the bad stuff. Just like in our intro to probiotics, back off a little bit and work your way up gradually. You can also add it to your smoothies, or make your own "healthy chocolates" by mixing the coconut oil with a little honey, cinnamon and cocoa powder. Mix well, pour into ice cube trays and keep in your fridge for a sweet treat.

Some cultures use unrefined coconut oil or cold pressed olive oil in lieu of toothpaste. It's called "oil pulling," and it is a highly effective way to rid your mouth of toxins. This is especially good when you feel a sore throat or other illness coming on. Swish it in your mouth for 10-20 minutes, as long as you can stand it, WITHOUT swallowing. You can spit it out and add more if you don't like swishing the guck around, but try to keep swishing and gargling as long as possible, then spit it out and wash it down the sink.

Try to eat fruit the first thing in the morning or between meals, at least 15 minutes before meals involving meat. Fruit (except apples) can sometimes interfere with how your body digests meat, so it's best to eat fruit on an empty stomach.

CHAPTER 7: Testosterone Boosting Recipes

This chapter covers some of the basics that you'll need to master to cook testosterone boosting meals the healthiest way possible – from scratch.

Bone Broth

Broth is the basis for many recipes, and it's one of the easiest, cheapest ways to add excellent nutrition to your diet. It's also a GAPS staple and a morning cup of broth will beat your morning cup of joe any day when it comes to producing testosterone. If you're on GAPS, you'll need to make plenty of broth every week so that you can drink a cup with every meal. But it also goes without saying that you can't have soup without broth, and it can also be used to make flavorful rice, beans, mashed potatoes, gravies and sauces.

One of the best habits you can get into is to roast a whole chicken every week, and then use those bones to make broth. It's also good to save the end pieces of your onions, garlic, celery and carrots in your fridge each week for the day when you make your broth. For a single man, one whole chicken can provide you with at least a few day's worth of lunches and dinners, and the broth will ensure nothing goes to waste.

If you don't want to use the broth right away, you can store it in glass jars in your refrigerator (let them cool a bit before sealing and putting in the fridge), and even put some in ice cube trays to keep in your freezer for seasoning dishes through the week.

A good batch of broth will thicken, and even begin to gel as it cools. If you've done really well at drawing collagen from the bones, your broth may even look like a jar of Jell-O in the fridge.

Ingredients:
- Bones

- End pieces of vegetables (use as many or as few as you have on hand): onion, green onion, garlic, celery, carrot, mushrooms, etc.

- Herbs: If you have them on hand, we love sage in chicken broth, and bay leaves and thyme in beef broth.

- Splash of apple cider vinegar (this helps draw out the nutrients from the bones)

- Sea salt

- Filtered water

A note about the bones: If you're using beef bones, you can reuse them up to a dozen times before discarding. Chicken bones degrade much quicker, so it's best to only use them once. However, if you're using the remains of a whole chicken, you can also add the gizzards to your broth for added nutritional value. It really doesn't change the taste.

Method:

1. If you have a slow cooker, put the bones (at least 3-4 good size beef bones, or the bones from a whole chicken), veggie pieces and herbs in the pot, then fill with water.

2. Add about a tablespoon of sea salt and a splash of apple cider vinegar, then replace the lid and turn on the slow cooker for 6-8 hours on medium low. It's easiest to do this before bed, then when you wake up you'll have fresh broth.

3. Once it's done, you simply strain the broth into a big pot, then add ingredients for soup, or pour into containers for storage in your refrigerator.

Stove Top Option

1. Get a big pot and add the bones, veggie pieces and herbs, fill with water and add a tablespoon of sea salt and a splash of apple cider vinegar.

2. Heat on high until it starts to boil, then skim any "scum" that may arise to the top (this is more common when using bones from conventionally raised animals), toss it out, reduce the heat to low, replace the lid, and let it simmer for 4-6 hours.

Obviously the downside to this method is that you don't want to go to sleep with something on your stove, and you absolutely can't leave the house. So if you don't have 4-6 hours that you plan on spending at home, you'll want to invest in a good slow cooker.

Roasted Whole Chicken

If you've ever bought a rotisserie chicken from the grocery store, you'll be happy to know that making one yourself is easy. All you need is a whole chicken, sea salt, pepper, about an hour, and you're in business. And again, it's a great habit to roast a whole chicken every week, then use the bones for broth and the meat for the rest of the week's meals and snacks.

Prep Time: 5 Minutes

Cook Time: 1 Hour

Ingredients:

- 1 Whole organic, free range chicken

- sea salt

- pepper

- dried thyme (optional)

The key to a great roasted chicken is to dry it thoroughly before putting it in the oven. This may seem counterintuitive to creating a tender and moist result, but trust me, it works.

Method:

1. Heat your oven to 450 degrees Fahrenheit. Rinse and thoroughly dry your bird with paper towels (then be sure to discard those towels promptly!).

2. Generously coat the chicken all over – top, bottom and sides, with sea salt, then sprinkle all over with pepper. The salt will help seal in the moisture, and having removed the moisture from the chicken skin, it will also help create a crisp and flavorful skin when done.

3. Place into a roasting pan or casserole dish, then place in the oven, once fully heated.

4. Set the timer for 50 minutes, then go prep your side dishes, salad, or start some homework.

5. At 50 minutes, check the chicken, as it should be close to done. Remove it from the oven, baste it with its own drippings, then sprinkle crushed thyme all over it.

6. Put it back in the oven for the remaining 10 minutes.

Now you can prep your salad, soup, or whatever else you're going to eat alongside your beautiful and scrumptious chicken! The best habit would be to peel all the chicken off the bones once you're done with the initial meal, then save the chicken in containers for the rest of the week, then throw the bones in your crock pot along with your veggie ends, water and sea salt to start a batch of chicken broth.

OPTION

If you can't get a whole chicken, or just prefer bone-in pieces, like whole legs, drumsticks, bone-in thighs, chicken breasts or wings, you can use the same method to roast the pieces, as well – as long as it's still on the bone with the skin on (skinless, boneless chicken can get too dry in the oven). Again, since we're using better quality chicken, we don't have to worry too much about fat content, as pastured animals have higher amounts of Omega 3 fat, which is exactly what we're looking for to boost our T levels.

1. Coat the pieces of chicken with your favorite spice blend, then arrange flat in a casserole dish or roasting pan and put in the oven as above.

2. Set the timer for about 30 minutes, then flip the pieces and roast the remaining 30 minutes.

3. For smaller pieces, like wings, you may need to flip at 20 minutes, and then only roast another 20 minutes, for a total of 40 minutes, not 60 like the bigger pieces.

I like these with homemade barbecue or teriyaki sauce.

Baked Potato - Brown Russets, Sweet Potatoes or Yams

It's not GAPS legal, but it's considered a "safe starch" if you're not suffering from digestive issues. It's also an easy and nutritious side for roasted chicken, and takes just about as long to cook.

Prep Time: 2 minutes
Cook Time: 45-55 minutes
Total Time: about an hour

Ingredients:
- 1 Organic potato of your choice per person
- Coconut or Avocado oil
- Sea salt

Method:

1. Pre-heat oven to 425 degrees Fahrenheit (or if roasting a chicken, it's OK to heat at 450)
2. Scrub potatoes thoroughly with water and trim away any blemishes.
3. Pat dry with a paper towel and rub skin with coconut or avocado oil.
4. Sprinkle oiled skin generously with sea salt and prick the potatoes with a fork to release steam as they bake.
5. Place on baking sheet and put in heated oven for 45-55 minutes, depending on the size, or until skin is dry and a fork can be inserted easily all the way into the center of the potato.

White Sauces and Gravies

A basic necessity for scratch cooking – especially when it comes to comfort foods – is mastering the "roux." It's really pretty simple; the key is not to walk away as it's cooking. The method is basically the same for making gravy, creamy soup base, or white sauce; you just adjust your ingredients and ratios according to the flavor and thickness you desire.

Ingredients
- 2-3 Tablespoons fatty meat drippings for gravy or creamy soup base (for white sauce, substitute with grass fed butter)
- 2-3 Tablespoons organic all-purpose flour (for grain free, replace with arrowroot at end)
- ½ teaspoon sea salt
- 1 cup broth (for white sauce, substitute milk or heavy cream)
- heavy cream (optional), according to desired thickness

Method:
1. In medium saucepan, melt butter over low heat, then slowly whisk in flour, sea salt and pepper until smooth
2. Continue to stir as you slowly stream in broth
3. Turn up heat to medium and bring to a boil, stirring constantly
4. Once it begins boiling, reduce heat to low and continue to stir until it's reached your desired thickness and consistency. Add sea salt and any other seasonings to taste.

For a cheesy sauce, follow instructions for white sauce and once the mixture begins boiling, remove from heat and stir in desired cheese (parmesan, cheddar, etc) 1 Tablespoon at a time until it melts in and reaches the desired taste and consistency. If it gets too hot, or if you fail to stir consistently, the elements will basically fall apart, so keep the heat low and stir!

Fermented Foods, Condiments & Salad Dressings

Fermented foods are pretty easy to make, incredibly good for the digestive system, and especially helpful for digesting meat.

Kefir and yogurt also serve as the basis for many dressings (and smoothies, too!), and incorporating them into your daily diet can completely transform your gut. Some people who have trouble tolerating dairy find they can tolerate cultured dairy, especially when homemade. They are amazingly simple to make – so much so that you'll wonder why anyone bothers with store-bought brands.

Making kefir and yogurt regularly can also help the habit of making other fermented foods. The liquid that separates from the kefir or yogurt (called whey) is full of healthy probiotics, and by putting just a tablespoon into a jar of ketchup, relish, mayonnaise, salsa, or other condiment – even those that are store bought – can transform a regular old condiment into a cultured addition to your meal. Just be sure to leave enough room in the jar to aid the fermentation process (about an inch from the top of the jar), cover lightly and leave at room temperature for 8-10 hours.

There are plenty of recipes for traditional fermented sides like sauerkraut and kimchi available online. But the basic technique is to simply shred cabbage and onions, then pound it for 10 or so minutes to get it to release as much of its own liquid as possible, then place in a large bowl or jar, add sea salt and any other spices or seasonings you like, add a Tablespoon or two of whey and allow it to ferment at room temperature for a few days. When the vegetables soften, you can transfer to the refrigerator and begin using.

My favorite is a combination of shredded red and green cabbage, onion, green onions, ginger and crushed red pepper. Play around and find your favorite, or culture your store bought condiments until you're ready to create your own.

Kefir

Yield: 3 Cups Kefir
Prep Time: 2 minutes
Fermentation Time: 8 hours

Ingredients:
- 3 Cups Whole Organic Milk (or Raw, if you can afford it)
- Kefir grains or Kefir starter, from your local health food store
- Fine mesh plastic strainer

If you can find kefir grains, they can literally last you forever. Even better, you can even find them for free, if you live near other health conscious foodies. A good way to find out is by asking your local natural foods co-op, or by looking for a local Weston A. Price Foundation (WAPF) Facebook group and join it. Make a post that you're trying to find some kefir grains and chances are someone will respond by giving you some of theirs. The WAPF groups are also a great resource for doing bulk buys of farm fresh foods like free range meats and dairy, grass fed butter, and other high quality foods.

Method:
1. If you start with grains, you simply put them in a big jar and pour the milk over them about ¾ of the way to the top of the jar. Place a napkin or towel over the top of the jar and let it sit for about 8 hours at room temperature. When done, it should have thickened and have somewhat of a chunky or curdled appearance, and it should also have a fermented smell, almost like beer.

2. Strain the kefir into another jar by using a plastic strainer (don't use metal or it may damage the kefir grains), then pour a little more milk over the grains – just enough to cover them – and store them in your refrigerator for later use. Kefir grains will stay good for months at a time. Or, if you're consuming your kefir daily (once you get on a kefir kick, you'll likely find many uses for it!) go ahead and make some more! The strained kefir can be stored in your refrigerator

for a couple of weeks at a time. But again, most likely it won't sit around that long.

3. If you start with kefir starter, you simply open the packet and stir the freeze dried starter into a jar of milk, again filling about ¾ of the way full. Then cover the jar with a napkin or towel and let it sit for about 8 hours at room temperature. No need to strain when it's done – it will be ready to drink or use in another recipe. Or store it in your refrigerator for later use. The downside to kefir starter is that it gets expensive, because you can't reuse it over and over again – and most likely you won't find any for free.

Homemade Yogurt

Yield: 3-4 cups yogurt

Prep Time: 10 minutes

Fermentation Time: 8 hours

Ingredients:

- ½ gallon Organic Milk (or Raw, if you can afford it)
- Freeze dried yogurt starter
- Fine mesh strainer and flour cloth towel

Method:

1. Pour the milk in a pot over high heat, but be careful that you DO NOT overheat it. You just want to bring it to lukewarm, to where you could still touch the outside of the pot and feel its warmth, but not burning hot. Immediately remove it from the burner and let it sit a few minutes to make sure it's not too warm.

2. As long as it's lukewarm and you can touch it, then pour about a cup of the warmed milk into a glass bowl. Open the packet of freeze dried yogurt starter and stir it in well with a plastic spoon. Once it's mixed in, then slowly stir in the remaining milk into the bowl. Cover with a towel, then find a nice warm spot to store it for the next 8 hours. It's a good idea to surround it with warm towels to keep it nice and warm to ensure it will ferment nicely.

3. If you have a crock pot with a low setting – or better yet, a Vita Clay crock pot that has a yogurt feature – you can pour the inoculated milk into the pot and set it on low for 6-8 hours.

4. Once the yogurt is done, it should appear thickened. If by chance it did not thicken, it's possible it was too cold during the fermentation period, or you may have put yogurt starter into milk that was too warm, which can kill the bacteria. But assuming the yogurt has thickened properly, then you'll want to strain out a bit of the whey (a yellowish liquid that's full of beneficial bacteria) to get the yogurt even thicker. I line a fine mesh strainer with a flour cloth (a very thin towel), pour in the yogurt and let it strain for about an hour.

You can strain for less time, but I like my yogurt nice and thick, like Greek yogurt. If you don't mind your yogurt somewhat runny, then strain it to your liking. Save the whey in a jar for later. You can reuse that whey to make more yogurt (about 2-3 Tablespoons to a ½ gallon milk) later, however at some point (probably after 2-3 batches), it will lose its strength and you will need to employ more freeze dried starter.

Store your thickened yogurt in the refrigerator for up to a week.

Probiotic Guacamole

Yield: 2 Cups
Prep Time: 3 Minutes
Ingredients:

- 2 ripe avocados

- 1 Tablespoon homemade yogurt

- Juice from 1 lime

- Sea salt, to taste

Method:
1. Peel, slice and mash avocados into medium size mixing bowl

2. Stir in yogurt and lime juice until fluffy

3. Add sea salt to taste

Spicy Fermented Salsa

Yield: 3 Cups
Prep Time: 15 minutes

Ingredients:
- 2 cans organic diced tomatoes
- 10-15 dried chili peppers (more for hot salsa, less for mild)
- 1 small yellow onion
- 2 cloves garlic
- ½ teaspoon raw honey
- 2 teaspoons cumin
- 2 teaspoons fresh lime juice
- handful fresh cilantro
- 2-3 teaspoons fresh whey
- sea salt, to taste

Method:
1. Pre-heat oven to 350 degrees Fahrenheit
2. Arrange dried chili peppers in a single layer on a baking sheet
3. Roast in oven for about 7 minutes, until slightly puffed (make sure you don't leave them in too long!)
4. Remove from the oven and set aside to cool.

5. Meanwhile, cut onion into quarters, peel garlic cloves and juice lime.
6. Once cool enough to handle, slice roasted peppers in half and remove the seeds.
7. Blend in food processor to desired consistency.
8. Transfer to container and stir in 2-3 teaspoons of whey, cover salsa and let sit at room temperature for 8-12 hours to culture. Cultured salsa will keep longer in your refrigerator, up to a few months even, and will continue to produce probiotics as it ages.

Homemade Mayonnaise

Many dressings use mayonnaise as a base, but as above, many bottle mayos incorporate bad ingredients and are high in Omega 6. It's not a bad idea to keep a jar of high quality avocado oil mayo in the fridge if you don't use it often. But if you use it enough, it's a good idea to get in the habit of making your own mayonnaise weekly.

Yield: 1 Cup Mayonnaise
Total Time: 5 minutes

Ingredients:

- 2 egg yolks – from the best quality (preferably pastured) eggs you can afford

- 1 tsp salt

- 1 tsp apple cider vinegar

- 1 cup olive oil, or avocado oil for a milder taste

Method:
The trick to mayonnaise is how you blend it. If you throw it all in at once you'll likely wind up with a runny mess. So it's important to start slowly and only add ingredients once it begins to thicken.

Homemade Barbecue Sauce

Prep Time: 2 minutes
Cook Time: 10 minutes
Total Time: 12 minutes

This is a very basic recipe for a quick BBQ sauce, but if you're a grill guy you should try adding your own spices and other ingredients to suit your taste buds. Whiskey, hot pepper sauce, and a touch of brown sugar might liven things up a bit.

Ingredients:
- 1 8-oz can organic tomato sauce (you can also use ketchup, but then you need to cut down on the honey)
- 1 teaspoon apple cider vinegar (or more, to taste)
- ¼ cup maple syrup or raw honey (or more, to taste – and only honey if on GAPS)
- 2 teaspoons liquid smoke
- 1 teaspoon dry mustard or 2 teaspoons Dijon mustard
- 2 teaspoons molasses (leave this out if on GAPS)
- sea salt, to taste

Method:
1. Pour all ingredients into a small pot over medium heat and bring to a mild boil.
2. Let simmer for about 10 minutes until it reduces a bit to form a thick consistency.
3. Taste and add more of any of the above ingredients to your liking.

Homemade Teriyaki Sauce

Prep Time: 2 minutes
Cook Time: 10 minutes
Total Time: 12 minutes

Ingredients:

- ¼ cup high quality fermented soy sauce (for GAPS replace with one part balsamic vinegar to one part beef broth)
- ¼ cup water
- 1 Tablespoon organic cornstarch (for GAPS replace with arrowroot and add at the end, not the beginning of the process)
- 4-5 Tablespoons raw honey
- 2 Tablespoons pineapple juice
- 4 Tablespoons crushed pineapple (optional)
- 1 clove garlic, peeled
- 1 teaspoon dry or grated fresh ginger

Method:

In a small pot, whisk soy sauce, water, and cornstarch together until smooth. Add minced garlic, ginger, honey, pineapple juice and crushed pineapple (if using) and bring to a boil. Reduce heat to medium, whisking constantly until it reaches desired thickness. If on GAPS and using arrowroot powder, you'll add that now and stir over low heat until it thickens. This has a higher sugar content, so do not leave unattended (or it will burn) and use sparingly!

Two-Minute Creamy Salad Dressing

Yield: 2 side salads
Total Time: 2 Minutes
Ingredients:

- 1 teaspoon Dijon Mustard

- 1 ½ Tablespoons mayonnaise

- 1 teaspoon raw honey

- pinch salt

- Fresh pepper, to taste

- 1 Tablespoon champagne vinegar

Method:

1. You can give this a whirl in your Magic Bullet or just whisk it by hand.

2. Blend all ingredients together until smooth, toss with greens and serve.

Fresh Ranch Dressing

This dressing is so simple and healthy that there is absolutely no reason to buy it in a jar ever again. The best thing about ranch is how versatile it is - when you need a snack, just grab some raw veggies and a bowl of ranch dressing and have at it! When you make it yourself, you get the benefits of the high quality ingredients full of nutrients you've mixed in with love - no chemicals, no soy, and since it's feeding your body healthy fats with probiotics, you don't have to worry about a "low fat" version.

Yield: 1 Cup Ranch Dressing
Total Time: 2 Minutes
Ingredients:

- ¾ cup kefir or buttermilk (shake well)

- ¼ cup homemade mayonnaise

- 1 teaspoon granulated garlic

- ½ teaspoon powdered onion

- ¼ teaspoon dried dill

- 3 teaspoons finely chopped fresh chives, cilantro or parsley (optional)
- sea salt and pepper to taste

Method:

1. Chop your herbs (if using) and measure your ingredients
2. Whisk together (or shake in a shaker jar) all ingredients and enjoy!

Option: To make this into a creamy blue cheese dressing, stir in about 1 heaping cup of crumbled blue cheese, plus about ¼ cup of homemade yogurt or sour cream.

Spicy Southwestern Chicken Salad

Yield: 4 Servings
Prep Time: 5 Minutes
Cook Time: 15 Minutes (if not using pre-roasted chicken)
Total Time: 5-20 Minutes

Ingredients:
- About a pound of chicken breasts or thighs (or peel off about ½ of your whole chicken, or roast 2-3 whole bone-in chicken legs – thighs and drumsticks)
- 2 stalks green onion
- ½ cup frozen organic corn kernels, thawed (leave out if on GAPS)
- ½ cup black beans (leave out if on GAPS)
- 1 avocado
- 1 jalapeño pepper (optional)
- 2 teaspoons dry or fresh chopped cilantro
- ½ teaspoon dry cayenne or chipotle pepper (or more if you like a kick)
- ½ teaspoon dry cumin
- 2 Tablespoons homemade ranch dressing

- 1 Tablespoon homemade mayonnaise
- ½ cup shredded cheddar, Monterey or pepper jack cheese

Method:

1. If you haven't already roasted a chicken, heat 1 Tablespoon coconut oil in a frying pan over medium heat, season the raw chicken breast or thighs with your favorite seasoning blend (we use sea salt, pepper, garlic, onion and paprika).

2. Cook for about 7 minutes on each side, until cooked all the way through. Then set the chicken aside to cool while you chop your vegetables and herbs.

3. To quickly thaw your corn kernels, pour into a small bowl of warm water and let sit for a few minutes, then strain.

4. When the chicken has cooled enough to handle, chop it to your desired bite size.

5. Then mix all ingredients in a big bowl, cover and store in your refrigerator for a few days.

6. Add freshly chopped tomato and chopped spinach or romaine lettuce when serving for added taste and nourishment!

Wild Salmon "Chop Chop" Salad

Yield: 2 Servings
Prep Time: 10 Minutes
Cook Time: 10 Minutes
Total Time: 20 Minutes

Ingredients
- ½ lb wild caught or sustainably farmed salmon
- 1 Tablespoon grass fed butter
- 1 bunch butter lettuce
- 1 bunch spinach
- 1 avocado
- 1 tomato
- ¼ red or yellow onion
- 1 red bell pepper
- 1 clove raw garlic, peeled
- ½ cup raw organic cheddar cheese
- sea salt, garlic and black pepper, to taste
- 2 Tablespoons of the 2-Minute Creamy or Poppyseed Dressing, or Balsamic Vinaigrette with a splash of lemon or lime juice

Method:
1. Pre-heat your oven to 400 degrees Fahrenheit and rinse the salmon filets.

2. Coat filets with grass fed butter, garlic powder, sea salt and black pepper and stick in the oven. Roast for 6-8 minutes. Set aside.

3. Chop and mince your greens and veggies – super fine onions and garlic, thumb size greens and veggies. Shred the cheese.

This salad will unfortunately not keep well in the refrigerator, so put it all together in a big bowl and enjoy right away!

Classic Chicken Noodle Soup

Yield: 4 Servings
Prep Time: 10-20 minutes
Cook Time: 20 minutes
Total Time: 30-40 minutes

Ingredients:
- 8 Cups chicken broth
- GAPS version: Spiralized noodles of a veggie of choice
- Non-GAPS version: Organic or gluten free pasta of your choosing
- Fresh veggies: Carrots, celery, onion, garlic
- Sage & thyme: Fresh or powdered. If fresh, 1-3 leaves, depending on the size of your pot, if powdered, 1-2 teaspoons, or to taste. If using fresh thyme, you can just toss the entire stem into the pot and remove it when done. No need to chop off the tiny leaves.
- Chicken: If you haven't roasted a chicken ahead of time, boneless chicken thighs are the quickest, cheapest option that won't add too much time to your prep.

Method:
1. Heat your broth to a simmer over medium heat.
2. While it's heating, chop your veggies into small chunks.
3. If you're chicken is not yet cooked, heat up a frying pan with a tablespoon of coconut oil, season your chicken well and fry for about 7-minutes per side, until browned and heated through. You can chop it in the pan with the tip of a bamboo cooking utensil, or move it to a cutting board to do a more thorough job.
4. If on GAPS, spiralize your veggie of choice into noodles
5. Add your chicken, noodles, veggies and sage to the broth and let it simmer for about 20 minutes. Add salt, pepper and sage/thyme to taste. If using spiralized noodles, add 3-5 minutes before soup is ready to eat.

Minestrone Soup

If you want minestrone soup and you don't have much time, you'll need to use a can of navy beans, rather than starting from dry beans. But if you have the time and are thinking ahead, the night before (or the morning) you want to use them, rinse about a cup of beans and remove any rocks that may have been packaged with them. Strain them and soak overnight. Or for the quick soak method, cover completely with water and bring to a boil, then remove from heat, cover and soak for 4-6 hours.

If you've done the soaking the night before, this would be a great recipe to throw in the crock pot in the morning before school or work, then enjoy in the evening with some fresh sourdough bread.

Prep Time: 10 minutes
Cook Time: 20 minutes (or an hour if starting with dry beans)
Total Time: 30 minutes to an hour

Ingredients:
- Broth
- 1 can diced tomatoes (plain or stewed to your liking – basil and garlic would be good here)
- 1 can or 1 cup dry navy beans
- Pasta (optional – omit if on GAPS)
- 2 carrots
- 1 stalk of celery
- 1 medium zucchini
- 2 cups spinach
- ½ onion
- 1 teaspoon dry thyme (or 2 stems fresh thyme)
- ½ teaspoon dry sage (or 2 leaves fresh sage)
- 2 bay leaves
- sea salt
- ground pepper

- parmesan cheese (optional for topping)

Method:

1. Heat your broth to a simmer over medium heat. If starting with dry beans, strain them, add to the broth and simmer for 30 minutes.

2. Chop your veggies, open your canned tomatoes and pasta, if using, and add everything to the pot.

3. Simmer for another 20-30 minutes, just enough to soften the veggies.

4. If using canned beans, strain and rinse them, then add everything to the pot at once and simmer for 20-30 minutes.

5. If using a slow cooker, fill the pot about ¾ full with broth, then add tomatoes, beans, carrots, celery, onion, thyme, sage, bay leaves and ½ teaspoon each of sea salt and pepper.

6. Cover and cook on low for 6-8 hours (or high for 3-4 hours).

7. About 30 minutes before the soup is done cooking, add the pasta, zucchini and spinach and cook another 20-30 minutes.

8. Once your soup is done, remove the bay leaves (and thyme stems, if you used fresh thyme), taste and add more sea salt and pepper to your liking. Pour into a bowl and top with fresh parmesan cheese.

Pan Fried Tilapia

High quality fish can be a tough one to find. Much of the fish you find in commercial grocery stores was farmed overseas in overcrowded, filthy waters, and fed diets that they do not naturally eat in the wild. Of the farmed fish varieties, tilapia is one of the worst. Wild caught can be a good choice, but pay attention to where they say the fish was caught. If that waterway is known for pollution (like a recent oil spill or nuclear catastrophe), stay away.

There are sources for sustainably farmed fish, but they're often pretty expensive. If you can find a good one, stick with it! (Currently, in our neck of the woods, Whole Foods is a trusted source for responsibly farmed fish that is reasonably priced.)

Prep Time: 3 minutes
Cook Time: 10 minutes
Total Time: 13 minutes

Ingredients:
- 4 filets tilapia
- 1 Tablespoon Grass fed butter
- Seasoning blend (garlic, onion, smoked paprika, sea salt and pepper)

Method:
1. Season filets generously with seasoning blend
2. Heat butter in skillet over medium high heat
3. Place filets in the skillet about ½" apart
4. Sauté for approximately 3-4 minutes per side, until golden brown

Enjoy with your favorite side dish – cooked cabbage & baked potato, broccoli & rice pilaf, GAPS fried rice, etc.

Oven Roasted Salmon

Salmon is full of healthy Omega 3 fats, but it's another tough one to find at a high quality and decent price. And in light of news that the GMO industry is looking to genetically modify salmon, you'll want to be even more cautious. Do your best to buy it from a trusted source, sustainably farmed or wild caught.

Prep Time: 15 minutes
Cook Time: 10-12 minutes
Total Time: 22 minutes

Ingredients:
- 1 lb wild salmon
- 1 Tablespoon grass fed butter
- 1 teaspoon granulated garlic
- ½ teaspoon dill
- sea salt, to taste
- pepper, to taste

Method:
1. Preheat oven to 450 degrees Fahrenheit
2. Rinse salmon filets and place on roasting pan to bring to room temperature
3. Coat each filet with butter
4. Sprinkle seasonings on each filet
5. Place in the oven and roast for 8-12 minutes, depending on the size and cut of the filets. Very thin filets, or end pieces, will cook faster, so be careful you don't dry them out.

Save any leftovers and use them the next day in an omelet or salad.

Cooked Cabbage

Yield: 4 servings

Prep Time: 5 minutes
Cook Time: 10 minutes
Total Time: 15 minutes

Ingredients:
- ½ head medium size cabbage

- 1 Tablespoon grass fed butter
- 1 teaspoon granulated garlic
- 4 Tablespoons broth
- sea salt, to taste
- pepper, to taste

Method:
1. Cut cabbage into bite size pieces
2. Heat butter in skillet over medium-high heat
3. Put cabbage into the butter and sprinkle with garlic, salt and pepper
4. Stir until all pieces are well coated in butter and seasonings, then pour in broth
5. Reduce heat to low, cover and simmer for 8-10 minutes

Do not overcook, unless you like mushy cabbage!

OPTION: Add onions and collards for more color and flavor
Method: slice onions, cabbage and collards into thin slices. Start by frying the onions until they begin to brown and caramelize. Then add the spinach and collards, and stir in seasonings. Add broth, cover and simmer on low for 10 minutes.

Buttered Carrots

Yield: 2 Servings

Prep Time: 3 minutes
Cook Time: 10-15 minutes
Total Time: 18 minutes

Ingredients:
- 6 large carrots
- 2 Tablespoons grass fed butter
- sea salt & pepper, to taste

Method:
1. Slice carrots into medallions
2. Heat butter in skillet over medium-high heat

3. Stir carrots into butter until well coated, add sea salt and pepper
4. Reduce heat to low, cover and simmer for 10-15 minutes, until they reach desired tenderness
5. Taste and add seasonings to your liking

OPTION: Add nutmeg, cinnamon, orange zest (or a splash of orange juice), and maple to sweeten it up.

Fresh Green Beans

Prep Time: 5 minutes
Cook Time: 10-15 minutes

Ingredients:
- 2 cups fresh green beans
- 1 Tablespoon coconut oil
- 2-3 Tablespoons broth
- Sea salt & pepper, to taste

Method:
1. Wash and trim ends off of green beans
2. Heat oil in skillet over medium-high heat
3. Stir green beans into butter until well coated, add broth, sea salt and pepper
4. Reduce heat to low, cover and simmer for about 7-10 minutes, until they're bright green and softened, yet still a bit crisp to bite.

Cheesy Broccoli

Yield: 2 Servings

Prep Time: 5 minutes
Cook Time: 10 minutes
Total Time: 15 minutes

Ingredients:
- 1 lb broccoli crowns
- 2 Tablespoons grass fed butter
- ¼ cup shredded raw milk cheese
- sea salt & pepper, to taste

Method:
1. Preheat oven to 400 degrees Fahrenheit
2. Wash broccoli and cut the florets into bite size pieces
3. Fill a pot ¼ of the way full with filtered water and bring to a boil
4. Fit a veggie steamer into the pot and fill with broccoli florets
5. Replace lid and steam for 4-7 minutes, testing at 4 minutes for desired tenderness (the fork should be able to ease into broccoli without it falling apart)
6. Remove steamer when broccoli is tender and place in oven proof dish
7. Coat with butter, season with salt & pepper, and sprinkle cheese over the top
8. Place in oven for 3-5 minutes, just enough to melt the cheese

Cashew Chicken

Yield: 4 Servings
Prep Time: 10 minutes
Cook Time: 13 minutes
Total Time: 23 minutes

Ingredients:
- 1 Tablespoon coconut oil
- 1 lb boneless skinless chicken breasts or thighs
- 1 large zucchini
- 2 red bell peppers
- ½ cup raw cashews
- green onions, as a topper (optional)
- ¼ cup sweet chili sauce (recipe below)
- 3 Tablespoons fermented soy sauce (if on GAPS, replace with one part balsamic vinegar to one part beef broth
- 1 Tablespoons sriracha (or your favorite hot sauce)
- 1 clove garlic
- Juice from 1 lime

1-Minute Sweet Chili Sauce

Ingredients:
- 2 fire roasted peppers (you can find these in a jar at most grocery stores)
- 1 small red chilli
- 2 large cloves of garlic, preferably roasted
- 1 teaspoon of freshly grated ginger
- 1 Tablespoon maple syrup (replace with raw honey if on GAPS)
- Juice from ½ a lime
- Salt and pepper, to taste

Method for Chili Sauce: Place all ingredients in your Magic Bullet blender and blend until smooth.

Method for stir fry:
1. Chop the chicken into bite size pieces.

2. On a separate cutting board (always cut raw meats on a separate cutting board from produce), slice zucchini into half moons, and chop the bell peppers into chunks or slices, whichever you prefer.

3. Fire up your wok or large frying pan with a Tablespoon coconut oil over medium heat and cook zucchini and peppers for about 3 minutes.

4. Add chicken and cook until golden brown, approximately 10 minutes.

5. While the chicken is cooking (be sure to stir it and flip it occasionally), put ¼ cups of the sweet chili sauce, soy sauce, sriracha, garlic and lime juice in a shaker jar and shake until combined.

6. Add the sauce to the chicken as it cooks.

7. When the chicken is cooked through, stir in the cashews until coated.

8. Top with green onions and serve over seasoned rice or GAPS cauliflower rice.

Dexterous D's Slow Ribs

Slow cooked ribs are so tender and delicious they fall off the bone. When you prepare them using beef broth, they're full of flavor. If you're a grill guy, you can carefully transfer them to a grill when they're done and baste the sauce on them for a few minutes over a flame.

Yield: 4 servings
Prep Time: 10 minutes
Cook Time: 20 minutes
Simmer Time: 3 hours

Ingredients:
- 2-3 lbs grass fed/pastured beef ribs
- 2 Tablespoons coconut oil
- Beef bone broth
- Seasoning blend (granulated garlic, onion powder, smoked paprika, sea salt, pepper)
- Homemade Barbecue Sauce (see Chapter 5 for recipe)

Method:
1. Pre-heat oven to 300 degrees Fahrenheit.
2. Season ribs with seasoning blend
3. In a dutch oven or deep cast iron skillet, sear the ribs in 2 Tablespoons coconut oil over medium-high heat until browned on all sides.
4. Pour broth over the ribs, filling pot to about ¼ full (ribs don't need to be completely submerged), cover with lid and put in the oven (or transfer to slow cooker and set on low).
5. Let simmer in the oven for 3-4 hours (or 6-8 hours if using slow cooker).
6. When done, remove ribs from heat, coat with barbecue sauce, and transfer to the grill or just enjoy as is.

Souletic Mama's Tacos

In my house we used to put practically anything in a tortilla and call it a taco. This, however, is our basic recipe for good old Americanized ground beef tacos. It's another good recipe to sneak in liver meat for a bigger dose of Testosterone boosting nutrients.

Yield: 6 Servings
Prep Time: 5 minutes
Cook Time: 20 minutes
Total Time: 25 minutes

Ingredients:
- 1 lb organic, pastured ground beef
- ¼ lb grass fed beef liver
- 1 Tablespoon avocado or coconut oil
- 1 small onion
- 1 bell pepper
- 3 cloves garlic
- 1 teaspoon cumin
- 1 teaspoon smoked paprika
- ½ teaspoon chipotle pepper
- 1 teaspoon oregano
- handful fresh cilantro
- 1 16-oz jar or can chopped tomatoes
- sea salt, to taste
- ½ teaspoon crushed red peppers (optional)
- Lime wedges, hot sauce, shredded lettuce, shredded cheese, salsa & guacamole

Method:
1. Chop onion and pepper into small bite size pieces, mince garlic, rinse and chop cilantro, shred lettuce and cheese. Set all aside.

2. Heat 1 Tablespoon oil in skillet over medium-high heat and add onions and bell peppers. Saute until onions become translucent, about 2 minutes.

3. Add ground beef and liver and stir in seasonings as you break the meat mixture into small chunks. Continue breaking it up into smaller chunks until it thoroughly browns.

4. Use the lid to strain off any excess oil from the pan (strain into a bowl and discard once cool).

5. Strain tomatoes, then stir them into the ground beef. Add minced garlic, crushed red peppers and let it stew for 3-5 minutes.

6. Serve with GAPS grain free tortillas, and top, cilantro, lettuce, cheese, salsa & guacamole.

QUICK FAJITAS OPTION: Cut the onions and peppers into longer strips and replace the ground beef with leftover roasted chicken, slow cooked rib meat (sauté veggies & seasonings with tomatoes, then add hand pulled chicken or beef) or vegetarian black beans until thoroughly heated.

GAPS Grain Free Tortillas

While they're not quite the same as a traditional flour tortilla, if you're on GAPS, these definitely do the trick. Make them for tacos, quesadillas, or even a flat bread sandwich and you begin to feel like you're eating "normal" again.

Yield: 6 "soft taco" size tortillas

Ingredients:
>1 cup egg whites (whites from approximately 6 eggs)
>¼ cup unsweetened coconut or almond milk (can also use kefir)
>¼ cup coconut flour
>½ teaspoon granulated garlic
>¼ teaspoon sea salt

Method:
1. In your Magic Bullet or food processor, combine all ingredients and blend well.
2. Let rest for 10 minutes to thicken.
3. Heat cast iron skillet over medium heat and oil lightly with coconut oil.
4. Pour batter into circle on skillet, tilting and rotating the skillet until the batter makes a thin pancake about 7-8" in diameter.
5. Let the batter cook for a minute or two, until the top of the tortilla doesn't look shiny and is not sticky to touch.
6. When the tortilla feels firm enough to flip, use a big wide pancake turner to flip onto the other side. Cook for another minute and it should be done.
7. Stack on a paper towel lined plate and enjoy with your favorite toppings.

Rice & Beans

You may be surprised to find rice and beans in a clean eating book, but this traditional dish is quite healthy when prepared right. It's also one of the most economical and filling dishes you can make on a regular basis. When you start with dry beans, properly preparing both the beans and the rice, it breaks down the starches and anti-nutrients so your body can break down the proteins and release energy from the carbohydrates over a longer time span. Cooking them in broth increases both the flavor and nutrients.

The bad news is, rice and beans are not allowed on the GAPS diet, because they still (even when properly soaked) take more effort to digest, with the exception of navy beans, lentils, and "faux" cauliflower rice (keep reading for that recipe). Once you've successfully completed the GAPS diet, you can reintroduce these healthy foods back into your diet (this was one of the first things I couldn't wait to eat when I came off of GAPS).

The method for making every variety of dry beans is essentially the same, the only difference being the amount of time it takes to yield a soft, edible bean.

Cooking with Dry Beans

Fresh beans are, of course, the best option, but unless you're buying from a really good farmers market, fresh beans are probably out of the budget or hard to find. So to get the best product and price, it's a good idea to buy beans from the bulk bin, as pre-bagged beans have often been sitting around in a warehouse or supermarket for more than a couple years, and old beans can be tough to soften (if at all). Bulk beans have a higher turnover, so you'll most likely get a fresher product. In all my years of cooking dry beans, however, I've only encountered one or two bags of old, hard beans. But I still prefer to buy from the bulk bin.

Approximately a pound of dry beans will cook up to 6 ½ cups of cooked beans. It's not a bad idea to cook an entire pound at once, then store whatever portion you can't eat this week in the freezer for later. You can store them in an airtight container (immersed in their cooking liquid) in the freezer for up to a year. I wouldn't let them sit in the refrigerator for longer than a week.

With all beans, be sure to start by rinsing and sorting out any rocks and sediment. Then soak them overnight (or for at least 8 hours) in water with a splash of apple cider vinegar. If you didn't think about it until the morning of, you can do the quick soak method of bringing them to boil in a pot of water, then removing from heat, covering and soaking for 4-6 hours. Be sure to always strain and rinse the beans when they're done soaking.

When you're ready to start cooking, start by heating a few tablespoons of coconut oil and sautéing a finely chopped onion and garlic (and any other herbs and seasonings you like) along with the beans for a few minutes. Then add enough broth to completely cover, plus a little over an inch to spare, and bring to a boil. If you don't have broth, you can use water, but then you'll just need to make sure you added enough onion, garlic, herbs, and seasonings to start with. If you like a meatier taste, add an organic ham hock or smoked turkey leg to the pot. A friend of mine always starts with a high quality bacon, then sautés the onions, garlic, bell peppers and pinto beans in the bacon grease, and they taste delicious.

At this point, you can either transfer to your slow cooker and set it at medium for about 4-6 hours, or you can leave it on the stovetop and occupy yourself somewhere nearby for the next few hours.

If the beans are small (i.e. navy beans) or fresh, your cooking time will be less, anywhere from 30-minutes for fresh beans, to an hour for dry small beans. If the beans are dry and large (i.e. kidney or garbanzo beans), your cooking time will be longer, up to 2 hours, or a couple more hours to thicken the bean liquid. If you're using broth, you shouldn't need to add salt, but if you're starting with water, wait to add salt until about ¾ of the way through the cooking process – about the time when you can smell beans and they can be cut through but are not yet soft. Adding salt too early can make the skins tough.

If you're using the beans for a salad, or some other purpose where you wouldn't want the cooking liquid involved, you can cook until the beans are soft and then strain off the liquid. Otherwise, if you're eating the beans as a dish on their own, you'll probably like a thicker bean broth, so you'll need to cook the beans for at least 3 hours, and then mash the beans with your spoon when they're soft enough to make the sauce thick and rich.

Vegetarian Southwestern Black Beans

Yield: 6 Servings
Prep Time: 30 minutes
Simmer Time: 4-5 hours

Ingredients:
- 1 pound dried black beans (for GAPS substitute with navy beans or black lentils and cut the simmer time down to 1-2 hours for navy beans, to 30 minutes for lentils)
- 1 small onion
- 2 garlic cloves, peeled
- 8-oz of your favorite salsa (optional – you can substitute with fresh chopped peppers, tomatoes and chilies)
- 1 teaspoon cumin
- 1 teaspoon dried chipotle pepper (optional)
- ½ cup coconut oil
- sea salt, to taste
- enough broth or water to cover the beans with about an inch to spare
- Optional toppings: shredded cheese, chopped tomatoes, avocados, cilantro and sour cream or homemade yogurt

Method:

Follow the instructions above for prepping the beans, finely chopping and sautéing the onion and garlic with your beans, then stirring in your cumin and chipotle pepper over medium heat. Add beef broth or water, along with 8-oz of your favorite salsa (this is optional, but if you're not cooking with broth you'll need it for more flavor). Bring to a boil, and after a few minutes, skim off any foam that rises to the surface. Add the oil, then reduce heat to low, cover and simmer on a stovetop for about 5 hours, until the beans are very soft and the liquid is thick and dark, or transfer to a slow cooker and set on medium for 6-8 hours.

Add sea salt & pepper to taste, then serve with shredded cheese, freshly chopped tomatoes, guacamole, salsa, chopped cilantro, and sour cream.

GAPS Friendly Green Chili

Yield: 6 Servings
Prep Time: 30 minutes
Simmer Time: 3-4 hours
Total Time: 3 ½ - 4 ½ hours

Ingredients:
- 1 pound dried navy beans
- 5 cups chicken broth
- 4 Tablespoons grass fed butter
- 2 Tablespoons garlic, peeled
- 1 small onion
- 2 cans fire roasted chopped green chilies
- 1 Tablespoon ground cumin
- 1 Tablespoon dried oregano
- 1-2 teaspoons ground black pepper
- pinch red pepper flakes (optional)
- ½ bunch cilantro leaves (or 2 Tablespoons dried cilantro)
- 2 cups shredded chicken (optional)
- Toppings (optional) sour cream, shredded cheese, chopped tomatoes & avocado, more fresh chopped cilantro

Method:

Follow the instructions above for prepping the beans, finely chopping and sautéing the finely chopped onion, garlic and green chilies in butter until the onion is translucent. Then add the beans and stir in the cumin, oregano and black pepper for a few minutes over medium heat. Add chicken broth and bring to a boil. After a few minutes, skim off any foam that rises to the surface. Add the shredded chicken (if using) and cilantro, then reduce heat to low, cover and simmer on a stovetop for about an hour to an hour and a half, until the beans are very soft and the liquid is thick, or transfer to a slow cooker and set on medium for 4-6 hours.

Add sea salt & pepper to taste, then serve topped with shredded cheese, sour cream, chopped tomato, avocado and more fresh chopped cilantro.

GAPS Friendly Red Chili

This is a great recipe for sneaking in some organ meat, if you dare. Start with just a small portion that you'll barely notice, then work your way up to more as you get used to the taste.

Yield: 6 Servings
Prep Time: 30 minutes
Simmer Time: 3-4 hours
Total Time: 3 ½ – 4 ½ hours

Ingredients:
- 1 pound dried navy beans
- 5 cups beef broth
- 1 pound grass fed ground beef
- ¼ pound grass fed beef liver
- 4 Tablespoons grass fed butter
- 2 Tablespoons garlic, peeled
- 1 small onion
- 1 red bell pepper
- 2 16-oz cans chopped tomatoes
- 1 Tablespoon ground cumin
- 1 Tablespoon dried chili powder
- 1 Teaspoon smoked paprika
- 1-2 teaspoons ground black pepper
- ¼ cup strong coffee
- pinch red pepper flakes (optional)
- Toppings (optional) sour cream, shredded cheese, chopped tomatoes & avocado, more fresh chopped cilantro

Method:
1. Follow the instructions above for prepping the beans, finely chopping and sautéing the chopped onion, pepper and garlic in butter over medium heat until the onion is translucent.

2. Add the beans and stir in the cumin, chili powder, paprika and black pepper for a few minutes over medium heat. Add broth and tomatoes and bring to a boil. After a few minutes, skim off any foam that rises to the surface. Reduce heat to low, cover and simmer on a stovetop for about an hour to an hour and a half, until the beans are very soft and the liquid is thick, or transfer to a slow cooker and set on medium for 4-6 hours.

3. About 30 minutes before you're ready to eat, in a medium skillet heat a Tablespoon of avocado oil over medium-high heat and add ground beef and liver, season with sea salt, pepper, smoked paprika, chili powder and cumin, and stir and chop until it is well done with a bit of a crust on it.

4. Add to the beans, along with coffee, red pepper flakes (if using), sea salt & pepper to taste, then let simmer for another 20 minutes. Serve topped with shredded cheese, sour cream, chopped tomato and avocado.

The Controversy Over Rice

There has been some controversy in the health food world over rice. For years, many people attributed brown rice as being the healthiest. But with the rise of the GAPS diet and more people coming to understand proper digestion, brown rice has taken a back seat once again due to how tough it can be to the digestive system. If you enjoy the chewiness of brown rice, or find it helps you with constipation, consume it occasionally, but make sure it is properly prepared. Brown rice must be soaked overnight with apple cider vinegar, or sprouted over 2-3 days before cooking.

The other issue with rice is that it has been found to contain measurable levels of arsenic. It is contained primarily in the outer layer (the brown husk), which is another reason to ease off the brown rice.

My rice of choice is white basmati rice grown in California. California grown rice has a lower arsenic content and the basmati version is lower on the glycemic index, meaning it doesn't convert quickly to sugar and thus releases energy slower. With white rice, you should always rinse it thoroughly (to wash off starch and arsenic residue), until the water runs almost clear, and if you have time, soak it in clean water for about 20 minutes, then rinse and strain one last time before cooking.

Seasoned White Basmati Rice

Yield: 3 Cups
Prep Time: 5 minutes
Cook Time: 20 minutes
Total Time: 25 minutes

Ingredients:
- 1 ½ cups organic white basmati rice
- 1 Tablespoon coconut oil
- 3 cups broth (or water)
- ½ onion (optional)
- 1 teaspoon garlic
- 1 teaspoon sea salt (omit if using broth)

Method:
1. After soaking and rinsing the rice, heat coconut oil in a medium sized pot
2. Mince the onion and garlic and sauté it in the pot for about 2 minutes
3. Add the rice and sauté for another 2-3 minutes
4. If using water, stir in the sea salt.
5. Slowly stir in the broth or water and bring to a boil.
6. Reduce heat to low, cover and simmer for 15-20 minutes, until rice is done.
7. Fluff with a fork and enjoy!

OPTION 1: Coconut Rice

Switch out half the water or broth for coconut milk. Add grated fresh ginger, cilantro or other herbs for more flavor.

OPTION 2: Parmesan Rice

Switch out one cup of the broth for a cup of crushed tomatoes. Then stir in ¼ cup of grated parmesan and chopped or dry basil, sage or thyme just before reducing heat and covering with the lid.

OPTION 3: Stir Fried Rice

Yield: 3 Cups
Prep Time: 5 minutes
Cook Time: 10 minutes | Total Time: 15 minutes

Ingredients:

- 3 cups cooked (leftover) organic white basmati rice
- 1 Tablespoon + 1 teaspoon coconut oil
- ½ onion
- 1 teaspoon garlic
- 1 bell pepper
- 2 stalks green onion
- ½ cup frozen peas
- 3 eggs
- fermented soy sauce (to taste)
- 1 Tablespoon sesame oil

Method:

1. Mince onions, garlic, bell peppers and green onion. Set green onion aside.
2. Heat a Tablespoon of coconut oil in a large frying pan or wok on medium heat, and add minced onion, garlic and bell peppers.
3. Add the rice and sauté for another 2-3 minutes.
4. Stir in the frozen peas and reduce heat to low.
5. Meanwhile, beat the eggs in a small bowl, then fry in a small frying pan greased with a little coconut oil.
6. Sprinkle the sesame oil and a little soy sauce on the rice mixture and taste. Add more if desired. When it's good, stir in the egg and diced green onion and serve.

GAPS Grain Free Rice

For rice lovers, the GAPS diet can be a challenge. This recipe got me through some of my rice and bean cravings!
Yield: 3 Cups

Prep Time: 10 minutes
Cook Time: 10 minutes | Total Time: 20 minutes

Ingredients:
- 1 Tablespoon coconut oil
- 1 large head of cauliflower
- 1 small onion
- 2 cloves garlic
- sea salt, to taste

Method:
1. Clean and grate the cauliflower into fine little shreds (that look like rice!).
2. Mince the onion and garlic and set aside in a bowl.
3. Heat coconut oil in a large frying pan or wok on High.
4. Add the grated cauliflower and stir constantly until it begins to brown, at least 3 minutes.
5. Stir in onions until they become translucent.
6. Top with navy beans seasoned to your liking for some GAPS style rice & beans!

GAPS Fried Rice

This is another great recipe for GAPS followers and Paleo enthusiasts.

Yield: 3 Cups

Prep Time: 10 minutes

Cook Time: 10 minutes | Total Time: 20 minutes

Ingredients:
- 1 Tablespoon coconut oil
- 1 large head of cauliflower
- 1 small onion
- 2 cloves garlic
- 1 red, yellow or green bell pepper
- 3 green onions
- ½ cup peas
- 3 eggs
- 2 teaspoons toasted sesame seed oil
- 2 Tablespoons apple cider vinegar

Method:
1. Clean and grate the cauliflower into fine little shreds.
2. Mince the onion, garlic, and bell peppers and set aside in a bowl.
3. Chop the green onions and set aside in another bowl.
4. Lightly scramble the eggs in a small frying pan and set aside.
5. In another bowl or jar, mix the sesame seed oil and ACV
6. Heat coconut oil in a large frying pan or wok on High.
7. Add the grated cauliflower and stir constantly until it begins to brown, at least 3 minutes. Stir in the mixture of toasted sesame oil and vinegar.
8. Stir in onions & peppers until they soften.
9. Stir in peas and taste test for more sesame oil or vinegar.

10. When the veggies are done to your liking, remove from heat and fold in the remaining egg and green onion.

Breakfast Foods

Athlete Pancakes

Although these are not GAPS legal, they are still quite a bit healthier than traditional pancakes. And if you purchase gluten free oats, for an added bonus they'll be gluten free!

Yield: 6 pancakes

Prep Time: 5 minutes
Cook Time: 7 minutes
Total Time: 12 minutes

Ingredients:
- ¼ cup organic whole oats
- ¼ cup homemade kefir or yogurt
- ½ scoop grass fed vanilla whey protein powder
- ½ cup egg whites
- 1 teaspoon raw honey (optional)
- 1 Tablespoon grass fed butter or coconut oil
- ½ banana, handful of blueberries or fruit (optional)

Method:
1. Blend all ingredients (except berries) in Magic Bullet or food processor. If adding berries, fold in after batter is blended.
2. Heat skillet with butter or coconut oil on medium-high heat.
3. Pour batter into skillet and cook until edges begin to brown and bubbles begin to surface around the center of the pancake.
4. Flip to other side and cook another minute or so, until both sides are golden brown.

OPTION: You can bake larger batches by pouring the batter into circles onto a baking sheet and bake in the oven at 350 degrees Fahrenheit, then save in the refrigerator or freezer and reheat as needed.

GAPS Grain Free Athlete Pancakes

Yield: 6 Pancakes
Prep Time: 3 minutes
Cook Time: 10 minutes
Total Time: 13 minutes

Ingredients:
- 1 cup cooked pumpkin or ripe banana
- ½ cup almond butter (or peanut butter)
- 4 pastured eggs
- 2 Tablespoons grass fed butter or coconut oil
- Raw honey, optional

Method:
1. Blend all ingredients in Magic Bullet or food processor.
2. Heat skillet with butter or coconut oil on medium-high heat.
3. Pour batter into skillet and cook until edges begin to brown.
4. When solid enough to flip, turn the pancake over and cook another minute or so, until both sides are golden brown.

Top with grass fed butter and raw honey

GAPS Grain Free Traditional Pancakes

Yield: 6 pancakes

Prep Time: 5 minutes
Rest Tome: 10 minutes
Cook Time: 10 minutes
Total Time: 25 minutes

Ingredients:
- 4 pastured eggs
- 3 Tablespoons coconut flour
- 3-4 Tablespoons Grass fed butter or coconut oil
- Raw honey, optional

Method:
1. Blend all ingredients in Magic Bullet or food processor.

2. Allow batter to thicken approximately 10 minutes.
3. Heat skillet with butter or coconut oil on medium-high heat.
4. Pour batter into skillet and cook until edges begin to brown.
5. When solid enough to flip, turn the pancake over and cook another minute or so, until both sides are golden brown.
6. Top with butter and raw honey

Dexterous D's Green Smoothie

Yield: 1 16-oz smoothie
Prep Time: 5 minutes
Clean Up Time: 5 minutes
Total Time: 10 minutes

Ingredients:
- 1 stalk celery
- 1 kale leaf and/or handful of spinach
- 1 small apple
- 1 slice pineapple
- 1 small slice ginger
- 1 small slice raw turmeric or 1 tsp dry turmeric
- 1 small banana
- 1 Tablespoon cold pressed olive oil or unrefined raw coconut oil
- Ice (optional)

Method:
1. Wash, peel, and slice produce
2. Put produce and oil in Ninja style blender and blend to desired consistency
3. Add ice and blend until ice is crushed to your liking

A note about green smoothies: Green smoothies can be hard on the digestive system when consumed too often. It's best to drink them no more than a few times a week, and be sure to add a high quality cold pressed oil, turmeric and ginger. If you're oxalate sensitive, you may need to avoid kale, spinach and other leafy greens and opt instead for celery, collards, cabbage, and lettuce, and rotate your greens to avoid developing food sensitivities.

Protein Smoothie

Yield: 1 16-oz smoothie

Prep Time: 5 minutes

Clean Up Time: 5 minutes
Total Time: 10 minutes

Ingredients:
- 1-2 bananas
- 2 Tablespoons nut butter
- 1 Tablespoon cocoa powder (leave out if on GAPS)
- 1 Tablespoon honey
- 1 cup homemade kefir or yogurt
- 1 Tablespoon raw unfiltered coconut oil

Method:
1. Put ingredients in Magic Bullet blender and blend to desired consistency

Oatmeal & Grits

If you're not on GAPS, oatmeal and/or grits can be a nutritious and filling breakfast. But to make them as healthy as possible, you should soak them overnight to break down their anti-nutrients and make sure your body can actually digest the nutrition they offer. It's extremely simple; you just need to get in the habit of thinking ahead.

Yield: 2 cups

Prep Time: 2 minutes
Rest Time: 8 hours
Cook Time: 5-20 minutes

Ingredients:
   1 cup whole oats or grits, or ½ cup steel cut oats
   2 cups filtered water
   ½ teaspoon sea salt
   splash apple cider vinegar

Method:
   1. The evening before breakfast, put all ingredients into your cooking pot, cover with a lid and let rest overnight.
   2. The morning of, heat the burner to medium and cook your oats or grits until creamy and soft, stirring occasionally. Whole oats or grits should be ready in 5 minutes or less, while steel cut oats will take up to 20 minutes to soften.
   3. When done, add a little milk, kefir or yogurt, and top with butter and honey, dried fruit or nuts, or cheese and hot sauce, if making savory grits.

Homemade Granola

If you're not on GAPS and miss the crunch and sweetness of a bowl of cereal, this homemade granola is the perfect alternative. Or pair it with a bowl of homemade Greek yogurt and sliced bananas for a high protein breakfast. To improve digestibility, the oats can and should be soaked prior to baking, but I have yet to master the art of soaked granola, so this is my current go-to recipe. Perhaps not optimal according to traditional standards, but certainly better than store bought commercial brands.

This is a basic recipe that you can use as your guide and then swap out your favorite dried fruits, nuts, seeds, and seasonings to your liking!

Yield: 3 cups

Prep Time: 5 minutes
Bake Time: 45 minutes
Total Time: 50 minutes

Ingredients:
  3 cups whole oats
  2 Tablespoons brown sugar
  ½ teaspoon ground cinnamon
  ¼ teaspoon sea salt
  ¼ cup raw honey
  2 Tablespoons pure maple syrup
  ¼ cup coconut oil
  1 teaspoon pure vanilla extract
  ½ cup shredded coconut
  ¼ cup flax seeds, pumpkin seeds or sunflower seeds
  ½ cup sliced almonds, chopped pecans, or walnuts

Method:

1. Pre-heat oven to 300 Degrees Fahrenheit.
2. In a large mixing bowl, combine oats, brown sugar, cinnamon, salt, coconut, seeds and almonds.
3. In a small saucepan, heat the honey and coconut oil over low heat until just melted and blended. Stir in vanilla.
4. Slowly stir in the melted mixture into the dry mixture until all oats, nuts and seeds are thoroughly coated.
5. Spread out onto a large baking sheet lined with parchment paper.

6. If you like your granola clumpy and crunchy, press the mixture down firmly.
7. Bake for 40-45 minutes, gently stirring every 15 minutes until the granola is golden brown and completely dry.
8. If adding dried fruit, add at the end, after removing from the oven.

Man Size Omelet

Once you get the hang of cooking omelets, the options are endless. These are particularly great when you're on the GAPS diet – eggs are such a staple on GAPS that a good omelet can serve as breakfast, lunch or dinner.

Yield: 1 Omelet

Prep Time: 5 minutes
Cook Time: 5 minutes
Total Time: 10 minutes

Ingredients:
- 3 eggs
- 1 green onion
- ½ raw sausage, removed from casing
- 2 Tablespoons spinach
- 2 mushrooms
- 1 Tablespoon parmesan cheese
- 1 Tablespoon cheddar cheese
- 1 Tablespoon grass fed butter
- sea salt & pepper, to taste
- Optional: ¼ teaspoon each granulated garlic, smoked paprika, dried turmeric, crushed red peppers, to add flavor and health benefits

Method:
1. Scramble eggs, shred cheeses, and slice veggies into small pieces. Set aside.
2. Melt butter in skillet over medium heat.
3. When butter starts to sizzle, squeeze sausage from casing into the pan, chopping into small pieces with the spatula as it cooks.
4. Once it's cooked through, add veggies and stir until they reached desired softness.
5. Add eggs and tilt pan around as the egg begins to cook.
6. Sprinkle with sea salt & pepper, add cheese.

7. Continue adjusting pan until egg is firm enough to fold in half.
8. Fold egg, then flip to other side and reduce heat to low, or turn heat off and wait as cheese melts and center of egg finishes cooking.

Hash Browns

Hash browns are not allowed on the GAPS diet (no potatoes whatsoever), and frying potatoes increases the amount of unhealthy acrylamides. So hash browns are not exactly on the world's healthiest foods list.

However, if you take a few important steps by soaking the potatoes and using a more stable oil, like coconut oil, ghee, or grass fed lard, you can rescue fried potatoes from the unhealthy category and keep them in the "in moderation" category.

Yield: 4 Servings

Ingredients:
- 4 Potatoes
- 4 Tablespoons coconut oil
- granulated garlic, sea salt, pepper, to taste

Method:
1. With a cheese grater or grater fitted food processor, shred potatoes into a bowl of cold water.
2. Let potatoes soak, completely submerged, in cold water for at least 20 minutes
3. Strain and rinse thoroughly, towel dry.
4. Heat oil in large skillet over medium-high heat.
5. When oil is hot, add potatoes in small batches.
6. Fry until edges are crisp and light golden brown, flip and repeat until all batches are done.

When your nutrition is right, your medicine cabinet will be your refrigerator. Keep these ingredients on hand at all times, and you'll be set against common ailments.

- Raw, unfiltered apple cider vinegar
- Onion
- Garlic
- Oregano oil
- Tea tree oil
- Unrefined and unfiltered coconut oil
- Cold pressed olive oil
- Baking soda

When you feel a cold coming on... drink a shot of apple cider vinegar at least 3X per day on an empty stomach. Increase broth and avoid sugar and grains until you feel better.

Sore throat... Gargle unrefined coconut oil or cold pressed olive oil for as long as you can tolerate, as often as needed. Be sure to spit out the oil; do not swallow. Increase broth and avoid sugar and grains until you feel better.

Acne attack... Avoid sugar and grains altogether. Increase probiotics, be sure to drink apple cider vinegar and plenty of water throughout the day. Wash face with apple cider vinegar, dry thoroughly and massage a small amount of coconut or olive oil onto face before bed.

Athlete's foot... Soak feet in warm water mixed with 1 cup of apple cider vinegar for at least 15 minutes. In between vinegar baths, treat infected area with tea tree oil.

Yeast infection... Soak infected area in warm water mixed with 1 cup of apple cider vinegar for at least 15 minutes 2-3 times a day.

Stomach Flu... Drink lightly carbonated water until you can hold down liquids. Then drink broth until you can tolerate more, then begin adding stewed vegetables. Increase probiotics.

Diarrhea... Increase probiotics immediately and drink plenty of broth and clear fluids. Firm/greenish bananas, cooked apples or applesauce (not raw), beets, cabbage, boiled potatoes, and plain white rice can help firm up stool.

Constipation... Increase probiotics immediately and drink plenty of broth and clear fluids. Exercise, eat cabbage soup, and consume helpful oils, such as fish oil or cod liver oil. Avoid pasteurized dairy, grains, starches and sugars.

Earache... Slice a small onion in half and put it in the oven at 300 degrees Fahrenheit for about 15 minutes. Remove from oven, wrap in a towel and strap it over your ear, then lay on your side and let the warmth of the onion sooth the ache. Keep it on as long as you can tolerate. The vapors will kill any bacteria that may be forming and thwart the rise of infection.

Hay fever/allergies... Consume locally sourced raw honey at least 2 weeks prior to allergy season to minimize allergic reactions to local allergens.

Note about antibiotics... Antibiotics should only be used as a last resort, as they kill all the good bacteria in your gut and disrupt healthy digestion. If you simply can't avoid them, you should spend the next few months increasing your probiotics, consuming as little sugar as possible, and drinking plenty of broth. Alternatives to antibiotics include raw garlic and oregano oil. Depending on the ailment, if you catch it early enough, you can likely avoid antibiotics simply by treating the infected area with plenty of garlic and/or oregano oil.

Additional Household Helpers

Most commercial household cleaners contain a plethora of chemicals, many of which may disrupt or mimic hormones. It's easy to minimize the use of harsh chemicals while still maintaining a clean household with just three natural substances.

Baking Soda: Scrub pots, pans, showers, and any other heavily soiled items. If you accidentally burn something onto the bottom of a pan or skillet, sprinkle plenty of baking soda and fill ¼ of the way with water, then bring to a boil on the stovetop. Reduce heat, cover and let sit for 15-20 minutes, then wipe the burnt food away like it never happened!

You can also wash your hair with baking soda, scrub dead skin from your feet, and use it to whiten your teeth.

Put ½ teaspoon of baking soda into a gallon of filtered water to make your own "alkaline" (pH balanced) drinking water.

White Vinegar: Dilute with water and use it to wipe down counter tops and clean windows. Once or twice a year, fill a plastic bag with straight vinegar and submerge shower heads for a couple of hours to kill bacteria.

Apple Cider Vinegar: In addition to the home remedies above, you can also use apple cider vinegar to unclog drains – first pour baking soda into the drain, then immediately follow with ACV. After washing your hair with baking soda, rinse thoroughly and condition your scalp with ACV.

Raw unfiltered ACV also makes a great toner for clear, healthy skin, especially if you suffer spots of skin discoloration.

ABOUT THE AUTHOR

Damon J Smith was born and raised in the California Bay Area town of Vallejo, where he spent a majority of his youth competing in various sports, including soccer, track, basketball, football, baseball, and BMX racing. After high school, he earned an athletic scholarship to pursue his goal of playing professional football at Utah State University. He completed four years at Utah State with a Bachelors Degree in MIS with an emphasis in computer science, and then earned the opportunity to play professional football with the Calgary Stampeders.

Upon sustaining a season ending injury with the Stampeders, Damon transitioned out of pro ball and into the business world, joining the engineering team at Intel Corporation. He then established a publishing company, Inspiring Minds Publications, and authored and published a sports motivation book titled, "Don't Stop the Swagger: Preparing the Mind, Body & Soul for Peak Performance." The book shares his athletic approach to developing talent through a strong work ethic, discipline and strategy, and applying that approach to all areas of life, specifically in the area of entrepreneurship.

An athlete at heart, he returned to the world of sport, only this time pursuing his lifelong passion for racing motocross. Though he had never ridden a motorcycle, he decided to put the premise of his book to action and see how far he could take it. By his third year of racing, Smith advanced to the competitive intermediate level. He began pursuing national level races, and qualified and competed at top amateur race in the world, the 2008 Loretta Lynn's National Motocross Championships. The following year he qualified and competed in the World Amateur Arena Cross Finals held at the MGM Grand Garden Arena in Las Vegas, NV, and by the end of his third year of racing, he set out to pass the rigorous qualification process required to advance to the pro level. Over the course of three months he traveled to Albuquerque, New Mexico; Salt Lake City, Utah; Reno, Nevada; Boise, Idaho and Spokane, Washington, competing against hundreds of other riders in an effort to earn his American Motorcycle Association (AMA) points and Professional License.

By the end of May, Damon earned his professional license and competed in select 2009, 2010, 2011, 2013 AMA supercross and motocross events.

Damon's competitive drive has always motivated him to pursue unconventional goals in life that require outstanding health and wellness. In 2012 he created Souletics®, a socially responsible technology company that develops products centered around health, wellness and peak performance strategy.

In April 2014, Damon was invited to speak about health and technology at the International Health, Wellness & Society Summit in Vancouver, Canada. In July 2014, he traveled to Rio de Janeiro, Brazil, following the World Cup to speak on race and the impact of sports on society at the International Sport & Society Conference.

The same year, Damon completed his 18th year as a Senior Physical Design Engineer (Mask Designer) with Intel Corporation. He has published six books, a documentary and fitness DVD, created a curriculum for underserved middle and high school students, incorporating health, wellness and mental preparation with STEM (science, technology, engineering and mathematics), as well as a 40-day transformational program, Soulpower.Academy.

Throughout all of his endeavors, Damon seeks to create a community of individuals who are nourished in mind, body and soul, and empowered to live life to its fullest.

For more mindset, health and wellness information, visit the
souletics.com

As we age, men's testosterone levels decline gradually, a phenomenon known as "andropause." It contributes to a decline in sex drive, decreased muscle mass, hair loss, weight gain, loss of energy, and sometimes moodiness. Although it's a natural part of aging, unhealthy aspects of today's modern culture may actually lower testosterone levels prematurely, leading to a condition called "hypogonadism."

In these circumstances, conventional medicine often calls for expensive testosterone replacement therapy in the form of pharmaceutical drugs. Many of these treatments, however, do have risks. Many of these "Low T" drugs have been linked to heart attacks, strokes, blood clots, and sudden death.

YOU HAVE ONE CHOICE:
CONTINUE LIFE IN A CAGE OR RETURN TO THE WILD.

Don't let the drug companies sell you on hormone replacement when you can increase your testosterone naturally, without negative side effects, and with all the benefits that accompany improved overall health.

If you suffer from fatigue, weight gain, moodiness, low sex drive, and low self confidence, this book is here to restore your vitality. Seize control of your life and...

GET ENERGIZED
LOSE WEIGHT
BUILD MUSCLE
INCREASE YOUR LIBIDO
and
GET YOUR SWAGGER BACK!

Real men get up when they're down. We figure things out. We get things done. Period. If you want to regain your manhood, the information you need is right here for you.

The only question you need to ask yourself is... will you be a LION, or prey?

Made in the USA
Columbia, SC
04 October 2024